Praise for *Embracing Change*

'Ever there was a book for its time, this is it. The sage insights and the very helpful guidance provided in this text should be of great benefit to those seeking to strengthen their resilience in the face of the many stresses we all face. Dr Barry has produced another book to be highly valued and incorporated into one's life'

Professor Larry Culpepper, Professor of Family Medicine, Boston University School of Medicine, USA

'Covid is a harbinger of accelerating change in the world that we all must learn to face. Harry Barry's book is a masterpiece of solid, highly readable, good sense, grounded in science, to help us learn to embrace this unpredictability'

Professor Ian Robertson, Professor Psychology, Trinity College Dublin and author of The Stress Test

'In *Embracing Change*, his most powerful book yet, Dr Harry Barry gently takes us through how life changes and we can adapt, with brilliant strategies and understanding, to everything life throws at us. How, by dealing with change, we can grow increasingly resilient and achieve great happiness in our lives. A magnificent book and a must read' *Cathy Kelly, author and UNICEF ambassador*

'This timely book from Dr Barry outlines insights and techniques with which we can develop the resilience we need to successfully move through change. It's the latest in a remarkable series that has shone a probing light into many facets of our mental health'

Dr Muiris Houston, Medical columnist with The Irish Times

'Without embracing change, it is difficult to thrive. To make beautiful new relationships, we might have to let go of old ones, to experience new wonders we might need to walk away from old patterns – I see now there is hope in change. We aren't built to hold on to everything we ever encounter. It's not easy to move on, to change and to adapt but *Embracing Change* has taught me that it is possible and a noble endeavour'

Stefanie Preissner, Sunday Independent Columnist, Presenter of the Podcast Basically . . .

'Once again Dr Harry Barry has written a most timely, practical and hugely helpful resource book. From his vast experience he shows us how, with his very practical, pragmatic blueprint, we can build up our resilience and learn how to respond rather than react to the challenges change throws at us, and improve and protect our mental health and wellbeing. This is a very powerful and empowering book'

Sr Stanislaus Kennedy, social campaigner, author and founder of Focus Ireland and the Sanctuary Meditation Centre

'Dr Barry has done it again! He has compiled simple but evidence-based techniques to mitigate against the stress we are all experiencing in these strange and turbulent times. Using his elegant step-by-step instructions, readers can develop the resilience needed to ward off anxiety and to improve their quality of life and relationships. From understanding the brain through to complex human interactions, Dr Barry's pragmatic advice will help everyone to build resilience and embrace change'

Professor Raymond W. Lam, Professor and BC Leadership Chair in Depression Research, University of British Columbia, Canada

'If you struggle with change, and let's face it who doesn't, grab yourself a copy of the excellent *Embracing Change*. Dr Harry Barry's fantastic framework gives you the skills to interrogate your own unhelpful reactions and replace them with resilient responses that liberate you from the confines of your comfort zone, leaving you free not only to survive, but to thrive in life and in the face of challenge. I really loved this book, needed more now than ever before'

Dr Sabina Brennan, health psychologist, neuroscientist and author of Beating Brain Fog

'*Embracing Change* is a must read. Not only is it a timely book but it is a toolkit, a book that captures the emotional journey that we all experience in our lives when dealing with change. Everyone will and can get something out of this book; those that embrace change and those that don't embrace change will see themselves in this book. This is a book I will share'

Helen Downes, CEO Shannon Chamber

'If ever there was a book for its time, this is it. The sage insights and very helpful guidance provided in this text should be of great benefit to those seeking to strengthen their resilience in the face of the many stresses we all face. It is broadly applicable but includes material focused on specific stages and challenges of life. Readers seeking to use this "bibliotherapy" independently, and those seeking to augment in person or teletherapy, should all find it highly accessible, engaging and, above all, immensely helpful. Dr Barry has produced another book to be highly valued and incorporated into one's life'

Professor Larry Culpepper, Professor of Family Medicine, Boston University School of Medicine, USA

'In this book Dr Barry teaches us how we should not fear change but learn to embrace it gracefully and with acceptance. He shows how sometimes it is possible to turn change into something positive. As with his previous books, this one is packed with practical and sensible tips that demystify change and reduce our fear'

Fiona O' Doherty, clinical psychologist

EMBRACING CHANGE

How to build resilience and
make change work for you

DR HARRY BARRY

S

First published in Great Britain in 2021 by Orion Spring
an imprint of The Orion Publishing Group Ltd
Carmelite House, 50 Victoria Embankment
London EC4Y 0DZ

An Hachette UK Company

1 3 5 7 9 10 8 6 4 2

A CIP catalogue record for this book is
available from the British Library.

ISBN (Trade Paperback) 978 1 4091 9989 2
ISBN (eBook) 978 1 4091 9990 8

Typeset by Input Data Services Ltd, Somerset

Printed and bound in Great Britain by Clays Ltd, Elcograf S.p.A.

MIX
Paper from

This book is dedicated to my beautiful wife and soulmate, Brenda, who has been my rock and intrepid travelling companion through the many and constantly changing peaks and troughs of life! 'Mo ghra, mo croi.' (My love, my heart.)

CONTENTS

PART SEVEN: SADNESS AND REGRET

INTRODUCTION

As I am writing this book, the world is grappling with two enormous challenges, both of which are blowing away our preconceived certainties as to how life should be. The first relates to climate change and how it is impacting severely on the lives of so many of our global citizens. The second relates to the Covid-19 world pandemic. At the heart of both lies the concept of change. We are being asked to reassess everything we believe in. Both issues are bringing change to the forefront of our lives, teaching us that much of what we base our lives on is both illusionary and self-deceptive. How much of our lives are built on shifting sands, rather than on solid foundations?

I have been interested in the world of change for over a decade. The more I worked with those struggling with mental-health problems, the more I recognized that episodes of major change in people's lives often underlie such difficulties. Those coming to see me were often 'stuck' and unable to move forward following such episodes. This was often putting intolerable pressure on their physical and mental health, leading to toxic stress, anxiety and depression. This led me to focus on developing insights and techniques to assist them, many of which I hope to share with you throughout this book.

I have also been interested, for at least a decade, in the importance of resilience in relation to our mental health and wellbeing. Increasingly it is seen as key to how we cope with, adapt to and manage change in its many and varied forms. In a previous book, *Emotional Resilience*, I explored the different skills that can help us improve in this crucial area of life. In this book, I hope to show you how, with the assistance of my five-question pragmatic blueprint, you, too, can learn how to build up resilience in your personal and working life. This is best done by learning how to apply this blueprint to the many situations that life will throw at you. I see this five-question blueprint as forming a framework for developing emotional resilience in real-life settings.

All of us struggle with change. It often challenges us, makes us anxious, depressed, frustrated or hurt, or frequently causes us to rail against both life and the world. But as the above world events are teaching us, change is inevitable, unrelenting and an integral part of human existence, whether we wish it to be the case or not. We do not require major world events, however, for change to wreak havoc in our everyday lives. In reality, each one of us is constantly having to change, adjust and adapt to much of what life throws at us, from birth to death. The good thing, however, is that all of us can learn to cope with change better. To become increasingly resilient and able to adapt to the challenges it can present.

Let's make this idea more personal. Do you find the concept of change challenging? Do you struggle to cope emotionally when some significant, often life-altering change occurs, sometimes without warning? It could be the sudden loss of a job, an unexpected illness, the death of someone close to you, the sudden breaking-up of a relationship – the list of potential causes are as varied as life itself. Have you come to fear and dread the prospect of 'yet more change', when faced with a series of expected or unexpected negative events? Does change make you anxious? Does it make you irritated or frustrated? Does it trigger unhealthy emotions of shame or guilt or depression? Does it make you feel hopeless or disempowered? Do you have the emotional resilience to manage these situations? These are important questions for each one of us to honestly answer, for so many of us struggle to deal with or manage change.

The aim of this book is to equip you with the pragmatic skills necessary to deal with change in whatever form it takes in your often hectic life. It will help you figure out how to make change work for you and teach you how to fully embrace it, adapt and move on. It will further help you understand the emotional, thinking and behavioural responses underlying change, and discover new techniques as to how best to manage it; how to become increasingly resilient and less disturbed about those periods in your life when change sweeps in and blows away all your 'certainties'. Each one of us has the innate capacity to grow and develop the skills necessary to achieve these objectives. By simply picking up this book, you are already taking that first crucial step in the right direction. You are wisely choosing to make yourself increasingly resilient, agile and adaptable, when such periods of change recur, in whatever form they take.

As a family doctor I have, over three decades, encountered countless examples of how life can throw up periods of change, often at key transitional points, such as entering college, having a first baby, the menopause and so on, and how such transitions can place enormous stress on our natural coping skills. I have also had to cope with the personal consequences of change in my own personal and professional life. Just because I am a professional, that does not shield me from the fickle hand of fate and how it can on occasion truly wreak havoc in my life if I, too, lack the insights and skills to manage it. I will share the knowledge gained over a lifetime of walking the walk with those of you encountering such phases.

In this book, we're first going to take a look at what change is and why we react to it in the way we do. If you can develop a good understanding of how and why *you* respond to change in specific ways, versus how *others* do so, you will find it easier to embrace and adapt to change.

We will look at how there are key periods of transitional change in all our lives. And then we'll explore the details of my groundbreaking five-question blueprint that will be the basis for managing any type of change in your life. Following on from this, we will look at how to use the blueprint in everyday scenarios by examining the six emotions people experience when faced with some sort of change, and delve into how you can use this blueprint to tackle that particular feeling. In the process, we will uncover some case studies that will be especially relevant to you.

I have chosen to approach this book by organizing it by emotions, because it has been my experience that the six feelings described are at the heart of *any* change. So, whatever it is that you're experiencing at such times, you can use the information and tools in this book to manage the situation you are experiencing in *your* life.

This book contains within it a resilience blueprint for life. It will introduce you to the immense power of pragmatism and how this can be seen as a shortcut to problem-solve so many of the difficulties that change can present to us. If you can learn to apply this pragmatic blueprint, it can be truly revelatory and you will discover much about yourself as a human being.

On your journey towards self-discovery you will meet myriad fellow travellers in the pages that follow. You may often see yourself in the stories that unfold and the life-crisis situations they encounter. I will discuss why they are struggling with changes in a specific situation and will demonstrate how our pragmatic blueprint assists them to manage such changes more effectively. I hope you will find some of the insights and techniques that I have honed over a lifetime life-transforming.

PART ONE

SETTING THE STAGE

1. The Many Faces of Change

The Inevitability of Change

A common quote – often incorrectly attributed to Mark Twain but actually paraphrased from a letter written by Benjamin Franklin – that 'the only two certainties in life are death and taxes', is one used regularly by myself when discussing the concept of 'control' with patients who attend my clinic with a diagnosis of anxiety. I sometimes wonder if a third strand should be added to this quote to include the word 'change'. For, like death and taxes, change is a constant human companion, from birth to death. Like it or not, change is going to challenge you, every step of your life's journey.

Yet none of us reflect on the reality or inevitability of change. How it can turn our lives upside down. How it has the potential to create emotional whirlwinds that can threaten to sweep us away. How difficult change can be unless we have developed the necessary skills to manage it. How change has been a reality for human beings since the beginning of time.

Change can best be described as moving from one state or situation to a new one. By definition, this suggests that something has been altered or transformed. And that, in practice, is what happens so often in life. You are sailing along merrily when 'that' phone call comes in and turns your life upside down.

I had a personal experience of this when, returning from a much-needed vacation, I received a phone call from my brother telling me that he had just been diagnosed with a terminal cancer and given six to eight weeks to live. Suddenly everything changed. I found myself having to face the reality of this unpredicted enormous change in both his personal and family life and indeed my own. Both of us had to travel different journeys in how we managed this change that was about to affect our lives and the lives of those we loved. I had to learn how to quickly adapt to a new reality. Three months later, he was no longer with us.

None of us are immune from the inexorable and constantly changing landscapes of life. Sometimes we will find ourselves at the summit of life, with all seemingly going well. At other times, often within a short period of being at the summit, we find ourselves struggling to survive in the valleys far below.

There is, however, the potential within all of us to cope with situations such as these. In 1859, Charles Darwin in his book *On the Origin of Species* suggested that we as human beings evolved through a long process of change and adaptation into who we are today. The key here is the word 'adapt'. For, as we will explore in detail later, the words 'change' and 'adapt' are like two sides of the same coin. To survive change, we must learn to adapt to it. This concept lies at the heart of this book.

There are three important messages here. Firstly, change is inevitable, a constant companion, accompanying us on our journey through life. Secondly, we must recognize and accept this reality. Thirdly, to survive and thrive, we must learn how to adjust or 'adapt' to change. When change comes, we have two options: to succumb to it and find ourselves blown around like a feather in the wind; or to discover new strengths within ourselves in order to manage such periods. The latter involves developing increased coping and resilience skills to assist us to survive, cope and eventually thrive.

The Speed of Change

As the Covid-19 pandemic demonstrated to the citizens of our world, change can sometimes present itself in a sudden, dramatic manner. Few would have predicted at the beginning of 2020 that within three months country after country would be on its knees, with deserted streets, areas in lockdown, flights grounded, borders closed, the sound of children playing muted, hospital systems overwhelmed, lives destroyed and the temporary collapse of the economic system as we knew it. How could all of this happen so quickly? This is not the way the modern world is expected to behave! How could a simple virus chop down all that we know, love and care about, with such ease, over such a short period of time?

There are many other examples of change, other than a viral pandemic entering our busy lives. It may be suddenly losing a job, developing an unexpected illness, losing your home, someone close to you dying prematurely. The list of potential causes of change is endless, and many of them will be familiar to every one of us.

Ultimately, what this pandemic, along with other unexpected events, teaches us is that life can literally 'change' overnight. Everything we believe to be 'certain' can be blown away in an instant. The world is now experiencing in macrocosm what human beings as individuals regularly experience on a personal basis in real life. When change occurs suddenly and dramatically, it can be extremely challenging for individuals, communities and even countries to adapt fast enough to unexpected situations that have arisen.

One of the reasons why we're so ill-equipped to deal with sudden change is because, in former times, change occurred in an evolutionary setting over hundreds of thousands, even millions of years. This allowed human beings to absorb changes slowly, giving us and other species time to adapt or adjust. One of the difficulties with technology and modern life is that we are now 'superseding' evolution by making changes and adaptations so fast that it is a struggle for us as a species to keep up with it. This pattern seems to be presenting itself in shorter and shorter cycles. Nowadays, what happened six months ago already seems outdated. Never has there been such a need for building up our resilience levels.

An issue concerning those of us who are interested in the mental health of our citizens is the manner in which modern life is accelerating change. Progress is relentlessly driving us forwards on what seems to be a path of potential self-destruction. The pace of life is inexorably accelerating for us all. There was a period when change occurred relatively slowly, over weeks, months, years or even decades. Once upon a time, we received a letter, considered its contents, then wrote back to the sender with our reply. All of this took weeks. Now we receive a text or email and there is an outcry if it is not replied to within an hour! This pattern of accelerated change, especially in the area of technology, has forced us to constantly 'react' to every new situation at almost breakneck speed. This puts immense pressure on our internal stress system and emotional brain, leading to increased levels of emotional distress and mental-health challenges. Most of us, for example, have 'brain fog' – where we struggle with cognitive processes affecting our attention, concentration and working memory – from trying to absorb constantly changing messages pouring in from social media and news-feed outlets. These control our lives, leaving little energy in the tank to cope with any form of unexpected significant change.

The Covid-19 pandemic, like so many life events, directly, if temporarily, stopped us in our tracks, forcing us as individuals to reassess how we are being swept along by the speed of modern life created by these 'progressive' changes. Hopefully one positive outcome may be a greater focus on what this is doing to our physical and mental health, and taking steps to challenge this situation. We cannot stop the speed of change, but we can perhaps discover how to manage it better in our own personal lives, with the application of sensible techniques.

The other great crisis facing our world and species lies at the opposite end of the spectrum and it perfectly encapsulates the other type of change we will all experience. Climate change, although seemingly accelerating at an increasingly fast rate in the past decade, is an example of how change, although taking place over a longer period of time and at this point expected, can still present us with significant challenges as to how best to adapt and cope with it. Like many expected and unexpected changes, there is no obvious, easy solution to this crisis. Furthermore, this sort of change similarly seems to be signalling to us that we need to alter our behaviour and slow down. Can we make the necessary changes and adaptations to save our planet and indeed ourselves and future generations? Only time will answer this question!

In our own lives, change can also take place over longer periods of time but still present us with significant challenges. Take, for example, the gradual adjustments one might have to make following retirement. Or having to adjust to the life-altering changes that the expected loss of a partner, parent or child might introduce into our lives.

We will be exploring many examples of both expected change and unexpected change throughout the book. Although you might anticipate one or the other to be easier to deal with, both can present different challenges and require different skills to cope with them. But it's important to recognize that whether a change is expected or unexpected has little to do with how you will react to it. We'll come back to this in more depth later on in the chapter.

Change Can be Positive

It's important to remember that there can be *positive* as well as negative aspects to change when it appears in our lives. Change frequently challenges us to reassess our current situation and identify new directions in which to travel. Sometimes such changes in direction may have dramatically positive effects on our lives. We learned much about ourselves, for example, during previous decades of economic depression. Many of us were forced to move away from different jobs or businesses, finding ourselves instead involved in more personally rewarding or fulfilling careers. So, change can present new opportunities for us as individuals to alter our lives for the better.

Gabriel's Story
Take Gabriel, a forty-four-year-old family man, who lost his job as a middle manager during the last economic downturn. Gabriel, in retrospect, realizes he has been miserable, going through the motions at work, dreading the long commutes, the boredom of his mundane job and the feeling that life was passing him by. As a result of losing his job, he is encouraged by his wife Eileen to do something creative. He decides on a pottery course.

This opens up a whole new world for Gabriel, who discovers his creative side, which had remained hidden for so much of his life. He throws himself into his new pastime. It soon becomes clear that he has a real talent. He gradually turns his pastime into a successful career, both financially and personally. Even when the economy recovers, Gabriel continues with his pottery, selling his work both locally and online. For him, change had altered his life in a truly positive, transformative manner. What initially seemed a negative turned into a positive opportunity.

There is an important message here: we must always stand back and seek out potential positives or opportunities from what may at first glance seem to be a disaster.

Apart from a simple career move, such as that experienced by Gabriel, change can also have transformative effects on our personal lives. We may find ourselves becoming increasingly resilient, discovering new insights about ourselves and our relationships with others. It can teach us to become more aware of our emotions and behaviours and how best to manage them. Change can also be a wonderful opportunity for personal growth. We can learn much about ourselves, how to identify our strengths and vulnerabilities and how to develop new insights and coping mechanisms. This book will assist you on this journey.

Why is Change So Challenging?

If you find change difficult to cope with, you're not alone. The first step to becoming a champion at managing change is to understand why you behave the way you do. As human beings, most of us will psychologically struggle with it. In the next section we'll be exploring the neuroscience behind change, since there are many reasons behind this struggle, but the principal one is our deep-seated human need for routine and structure in our lives, despite on occasion bemoaning both.

We all develop patterns and become comfortable with them. At each stage of our lives, human beings fall into set routines and patterns of behaviour. We build a protective structure around ourselves, making us feel safe and secure. We rarely notice or comment about these structures, but simply learn to accept them as 'normal' for us. This concept also underlies the world of anxiety, where we erroneously believe that we should be in absolute control of our lives and struggle to cope when this demand cannot be met.

Change fundamentally challenges the safe and secure structures which we have built up around ourselves, in the form of these routines and patterns of behaviour. If change is sudden or dramatic, these seemingly 'solid' foundations and structures can be blown away with almost casual indifference, thus destroying our carefully organized world.

When a significant personal change occurs in your life, especially one that is negative or distressing, routines and structures can also be easily cast aside, exposing the reality that life is not as safe and secure as you had previously believed. A common example of such a change might be when a young child becomes suddenly ill with meningitis or pneumonia. Suddenly the lives of the parents involved are turned upside down, with all their attention switched away from their everyday routines to a life-and-death bedside vigil with their acutely ill child. Change challenges us emotionally and this in turn may force us to behave differently.

It may also seriously challenge our beliefs about ourselves and the world. We will be discussing this in greater detail later.

Another reality is that all of us hate to see our routines and structures altered or changed, unless we believe that this change emanates from ourselves. We like to feel that 'we' are in charge of events in our lives. It can come as an unwelcome shock when matters are taken out of our hands by life itself, as so often happens. This can cause us intense disturbance and discomfort, and as human beings discomfort is something we prefer to avoid. Change, by uprooting our normal routines and patterns, can make us feel less safe, less 'in control', which makes us afraid for ourselves and those we love.

The challenge for you personally if you truly wish to embrace change, however challenging this may seem on occasion, is to learn about yourself. What are the routines and patterns and structures that you have wrapped around yourself? How do you respond emotionally and otherwise when those safe, secure bastions are challenged and ruptured by some stressful change emerging into your life?

Change will always be challenging and difficult. But we can develop new ways of understanding and behaving which can make this challenge easier to surmount. In the process we can grow and develop as human beings. I firmly believe that many of us are confined within the structures that we place around ourselves, like caterpillars in a pupa. If we, like the caterpillar, can learn how to break out of this structure, we can become the beautiful free butterflies that all of us truly are. That is our challenge in this book. To set you free!

The Neuroscience of Change

Let's now explore what is going on from a neuroscience perspective. There are three significant players in the brain, which are key to how we understand change. The first structure, situated at the front of the brain, is called the prefrontal cortex (PFC), and is the thinking, sensible, rational (to a point), problem-solving part of the brain.

The second structure, situated in the middle of the brain, is called the limbic system. Alongside monitoring vital bodily functions, one of its primary functions is to oversee our emotional world, which is why it is frequently referred to as the emotional brain. A key player here is the amygdala. The amygdala is seen as the mother and father of most of our emotions, especially sadness, depression, anxiety, panic, anger, frustration, rage and so on. The amygdala will also store the memory of our emotional reactions to change or any other occurrence in our lives. It is critically important to realize that your amygdala is also the boss of your stress system. This explains why change 'stresses us out' physically as well as psychologically. We are truly holistic.

A third key brain structure when discussing change is called the basal ganglia, which is also part of the limbic system. When we begin to develop any new task, such as learning to drive a car, for example, the brain usually employs the PFC, especially on the right side, to engage firstly in the task. There is also plenty of input from the limbic system or our emotional brain, especially from the amygdala, as there are usually plenty of emotions swilling around when we apply ourselves to a new task. You probably recall the emotions of fear and anxiety that accompanied your first few driving lessons!

When you have, over time, through constant practice, achieved your objective and become accomplished at the task, responsibility shifts to the left side of the brain. The brain also shifts future responsibility for carrying out the task (in this case, driving the car) to other parts of the brain such as the basal ganglia. This is a lower-level structure that uses up less energy and allows us to complete the task almost unconsciously. We get into the car and just drive, without having to 'think' about it.

When we encounter significant change in our lives, we initially engage the right PFC and amygdala in particular as we try to come to the terms with the rational and emotional consequences that can often emanate from it. Over time, if we learn to adapt to change, the brain will be able to shift attention to newer challenges and allow more low-key structures to manage our new behaviours.

The brain dislikes change as it challenges the homeostatic *status quo*, which it craves. There are practical reasons as to why it resists change. Change will often require precious cognitive and energy reserves, which the brain deems essential. It therefore avoids or resists changing the *status quo*, unless absolutely forced to do so. This is why we all find it so difficult to change our habits or behaviours. There is a cerebral as well as psychological cost to making the necessary changes.

We also tend to respond to change emotionally, which many of us struggle with. Rather than coming to terms with such emotions, our natural response is to want to return to where we were. Life, however, does not remain static, it is relentlessly and inexorably moving on and changing. From the brain's perspective, emotions also exhaust valuable reserves, which is why it finds change exhausting.

To cope with change, we must recognize and accept the role of our emotional brain, especially the amygdala. Sometimes we may have to stay with these emotions for some time before we are ready to move on to explore matters cognitively. A classic example of this might be coping with the loss of a loved one. We must first recognize and absorb the emotions of grief and only then can we move on to explore the practical issues which such a change in our lives might create. It will be our PFC that assists us in dealing with the latter.

Later we will look at how you can learn new techniques to assist both you and your brain to overcome your natural psychological and brain resistance to change. Over time, with these techniques you can learn how to calm down your amygdala and reset your PFC.

Before leaving the neuroscience of change, it is important to also realize that the human brain has developed a unique way of dealing with the constant barrage of changes that life throws our way. The brain allows us to increase or decrease key connections between individual neurons and, through this facility, to alter key neural pathways in the brain. We call this facility 'neuroplasticity'. It is hard to believe, but this process is going on continuously every moment of the day. This allows the brain to adapt to new circumstances in a reactive manner. If change is short-lived and temporary, the brain's response will behave accordingly. But if change is significant, or life-transforming, then it will take longer periods, often weeks, months or even years, to change our connections and neural pathways to adapt long term.

This knowledge is essential as it demonstrates that your capacity to cope with and adapt to change is not something that you can develop overnight. It takes time to develop and embed into your psyche and brain the necessary insights and techniques which will allow you to manage change, in whatever form it takes in your life. The good news is that once you have developed such techniques, you will be increasingly resilient and capable of embracing change into the future.

We also know that the brain is constantly changing from birth to death. We can divide this process into three periods:

1. The Developing Brain – the period between birth and the age of thirty. This includes the Adolescent Brain, which covers the phase between thirteen and thirty. During this latter period, the brain is gradually 'pruning' and reorganizing its connections and pathways to make them as efficient and effective as possible.
2. The Mature Brain – the period between thirty and sixty-five. This is the phase where the brain gradually becomes increasingly efficient, learning how to pragmatically mould our emotional and logical brains together to solve whatever problems or issues present themselves.
3. The Ageing Brain – the period from sixty-five to the end of our lives. This is the phase where the brain slowly, over decades, begins to shed or reduce connections and neurons. Thankfully, with our modern understanding of the importance of exercise, nutrition and social connections, we can develop techniques to slow down this process.

It is important to realize that our brain is gradually changing, just as our own lives are altering and transforming.

The Three Phases of Life

It is also useful to divide our lives into three phases, which in many ways mirror the three ages of the brain. Let's explore them and mention especially some common transitional periods where change can present itself, often challenging us to the core.

1.   The Early Decades – the first three decades of life. We move from children (birth to eighteen) to young adulthood (eighteen to twenty-five), slowly moving to full maturity as human beings by thirty. Key transitional periods during this phase are early to mid-adolescence; entering secondary school; entering tertiary education; beginning a new job; breakdown of first relationship; arrival of first baby; coping with the arrival of mental-health difficulties for the first time; and so on.

2.   The Middle Decades – between thirty and sixty-five. This constitutes the bulk of our lives. We are fully mature adults at the peak of our careers and lives. This is the period when we form long-term relationships; may begin and rear families; cope with increasing work pressures as we advance in our careers; have to assist ageing parents as they encounter increasing frailty; cope with the loss of parents or siblings; deal with issues associated with emerging adolescents and young adults; manage the empty-nest syndrome as our children move on into their new lives; and so on.

3.   The Later Decades – from sixty-five to the end of our lives. I often describe this phase as a 'period of loss' and it can on occasion be the most challenging. Many of the transitional periods of change which we can encounter during this phase will involve the loss of things that are dear to us. Loss can be painful and extremely challenging. This can be a phase where we have to encounter retirement; the loss of siblings, adult children, loved

ones or close friends; the gradual loss over decades of elements of our physical health; the challenges of loneliness; financial restraints; illness in its many forms; the loss of mobility and independence; and so on.

It is essential to emphasize that all three phases of life will be filled with wonderful moments and periods of joy, happiness and personal fulfilment. There will be times when we are up on top of the mountain and all is well. We will experience positive change where we can grow and develop as human beings.

While often in life change can present an exciting challenge, sometimes we may find ourselves down in the valleys of life, where change brings us to our knees, emotionally shattering our previously calm and joyous existence. Some of the transitional periods noted above can introduce such periods into our lives. Whether you lose your job at twenty or sixty-five years old, however, it is not especially helpful to manage change from an age perspective. Instead, at the core of this work, and what will make this resilience blueprint more personal to you, is looking at your personal emotional responses to any given change.

The Emotional and Behavioural Consequences of Change

Emotional Consequences

Earlier we discussed how the brain reacts to change and we touched on how emotional our brains are. Emotions are powerfully intense feelings or sensations that can be triggered by conscious or unconscious events. Emotions can be positive or negative, and healthy or unhealthy.

Positive emotions include joy, happiness, pleasure, love, awe, trust, contentment and peacefulness. We call these emotions positive because they make us feel good about ourselves and give us a sense of wellbeing.

There are also healthy negative emotions that help us cope with the many difficulties life throws at us, such as loss. A healthy negative emotion such as sadness is still uncomfortable, but it is helpful as it allows us to sit with and attempt to come to terms with some loss in our lives.

Unhealthy negative emotions, however, often impede us in dealing with such difficulties. We classify depression as an unhealthy negative emotion, for example, as it makes us feel bad about ourselves, which may result in unhealthy behaviours such as isolating ourselves from other people. A major change such as the arrival of a newborn baby into a house is usually associated with healthy positive emotions such as joy or happiness.

This distinction between healthy and unhealthy emotions is important. With healthy emotions, we can develop new ways to move forward following the change, as in the case of sadness following the loss of someone close to us. However, unhealthy negative emotions can suffocate our capacity to move on and lock us into negative downward spirals.

For instance, if I, as the mother of a newborn baby, believe erroneously that I am not coping as well as others in my situation, I may experience the negative unhealthy emotion of depression, which may lead me to become significantly emotionally distressed. If this is something you are experiencing right now, read on, as we will be exploring this scenario later.

In Parts Two to Seven of this book, we will look at the six most common unhealthy negative emotions we face when encountering change and what tools we can use to manage each accordingly.

It is important from the beginning to self-identify your personal emotional response to a stressful period of change in your life, as it is key in finding your path out of the maze. This is why we often call emotions 'signposts' into the inner world of ourselves, which is hidden to those on the outside.

It is also important to realize that our emotions can trigger physical symptoms and that these, too, can be distressing. If sad, I may shed copious tears. If anxious, I may notice that I complain of fatigue, my stomach feeling as if it's in knots, feeling wired, tension headaches or teeth-grinding at night. If panicking, I may find my heart pounding, and that I am shaking, sweating, hyper-ventilating, etc. All of these physical sensations are caused by my emotional brain activating my internal stress system.

Behavioural Consequence

Behaviour is best defined as what we do and is usually our re-sponse to some emotion that has been triggered by some event in our internal or external environment. Our behaviours are useful in assisting us to pinpoint our emotions if we are struggling to identify them. Nowhere are our behaviours more relevant as when we are coping with significant periods of change.

One of the first casualties following sudden unexpected change, such as the sudden breakdown of a long-term relation-ship, is usually our lifestyle behaviours. How often, when anxious or depressed at such times, do we eat poorly, cease exercising, get insufficient sleep, drink too much, spend too much time on social media or allow our routines and structures to fall apart?

Other behavioural consequences of change can relate more to safety or avoidant behaviours. A great example of this was the panic-buying of toilet rolls and widespread amassing of months' worth of food at the beginning of the Covid-19 pandemic, much of which had to be subsequently thrown away. This was to satisfy our initial, if understandable, emotion of panic.

The most serious behavioural consequence of change relates to the decision by some people to self-harm. The change is just too overwhelming, swamping them emotionally and cognitively, leading in turn to this profoundly negative behaviour. This is tragic, as change is as much about how we view it as it is about the change itself. Assisting people to reassess how they are thinking and feeling about the source of their distressing change can lead to them moving away from such destructive behaviours. The most tragic example of this is where a family member such as a parent or sibling decides to take their own life when they are overcome by the struggle to cope with the changes in their life triggered by the overwhelming loss of a loved one to suicide.

Human beings are often completely irrational when it comes to their thinking patterns, and nowhere does this come to the surface more than when faced with overwhelming change in our lives. This in turn leads to many of the negative emotions and self-destructive behaviours that can cause us so much distress at such times.

Yet when faced with change, some of us seem to cope better with new situations while others really struggle. Some respond with healthy emotions, but many do not. Clearly there is some missing link underlying these differences in response, namely our thoughts.

2. Embracing Change

The Role of Our Thoughts in Coping with Change

The missing link between the event that caused the change in our lives and how we respond emotionally and behaviourally turns out to be our thoughts, or how we choose to think about such events. This interrelationship has been known for centuries. The Greek Stoic philosopher Epictetus (50–138 AD) stated that 'men are disturbed not by things but the view which they take of them'. This philosophical insight underlies the basis of Cognitive Behaviour Therapy, or CBT. The person credited with transforming the way in which we linked thoughts, emotions and behaviours together was Albert Ellis, arguably one of the greatest psychotherapists of the last hundred years. Although I do not plan to specifically use CBT techniques throughout this book, we will draw on some of his ideas.

Thoughts are best defined as the words, images, ideas, memories, beliefs and concepts that flow in and out of your conscious mind. Ellis believed that our interpretation of events (or how we 'think' about them), which can cause us so much emotional pain, was based on simple inbuilt belief systems that we developed as human beings mainly due to our experiences in childhood. He called these belief systems Rational and Irrational Beliefs.

He believed that all of us develop such beliefs, which we pick up like viruses when passing through childhood, adolescence and young adult life. Rational beliefs are sensible and logical and lead to healthy negative emotions such as sadness. Irrational beliefs, on the other hand, are destructive, unhelpful and often completely illogical and lead to unhealthy negative emotions such as anxiety, frustration or depression.

Our individual responses to, for example, being left on our own following the sudden death of a long-term partner relates to how we 'thought' about it. This in turn relates back to whether this significant change in our lives triggered our rational or irrational beliefs. If it is the former, we might have been sad or concerned about the situation. If the latter, we might be angry, frustrated, anxious or depressed about it.

If, for example, I am struggling with the belief that I will never be able to cope with this new situation in which I find myself, following such a loss, convincing myself that it will be endless and awful, then my emotion may be anxiety. If I am demanding that this situation should not be happening, then my emotion might be frustration. If I was not at home when my loved one died suddenly, my emotion might be guilt. If I am desperately missing the presence of the person I have loved all my life and struggling to accept that they are not returning, my emotion might be simply sadness. Depending on how each one of us 'thought about' their changed circumstances following such a loss, this would affect how we would cope emotionally or behaviourally.

This insight is absolutely vital. If we can learn to quickly identify how we are responding emotionally to a sudden change in our lives, this can signpost whether our thinking about the event is helpful or not. So it will be our thinking, or interpretation of what has happened to us, which will determine how well we will or will not cope emotionally or behaviourally with change. If we can learn some insights and techniques as to how best to adjust or adapt our 'thinking' about situations that cause change, it becomes easier to manage them. We can learn how to embrace rather than fear change.

Those interested in exploring the world of CBT in greater detail are advised to refer to some of my previous books. In this book, I plan to use some of the above insights into how our thoughts, emotions and behaviour are all linked together, but combine them under one heading – pragmatism.

I have always believed that our modern obsession with the importance of positive thinking has frequently prevented us from focusing on what really matters, namely realistic or pragmatic thinking. It is not that I am against the concept of positive versus negative thinking, it is the assumption that either can really make any significant difference to the final result in every case. If I have a seriously and rapidly growing cancer, for example, no amount of positive thinking can change the eventual outcome.

Real life is not a rosy place where boosting positive thinking (which may be of assistance in some situations) will inevitably ensure a desired result. Rather, it is a place where pragmatism rules supreme. So, what is pragmatism?

What is Pragmatism?

Pragmatism is a life skill whereby we become adept at quickly analysing problematic situations with a view to finding and putting into practice the most effective solutions. It is first and foremost about being practical. It teaches us how to carve through fixed or unhelpful thinking or behavioural patterns to achieve this objective. Pragmatists become experts at finding the 'short cut' to how best to deal with practical everyday difficulties. Pragmatism also involves taking the world as we find it, not as we would like it to be.

We can immediately see how pragmatism fits neatly into our discussion on change. Change, as we have seen already, is inevitable – an inexorable part of our existence, a constant challenge and something that has the power to make or break us. Pragmatism allows us to smoothly navigate a safe passage through difficult periods of change in our lives.

Before exploring how you too can develop the skill of pragmatism, let's discuss the importance of using simply pen and paper when attempting to analyse and problem-solve difficulties which some significant change may be presenting in your life.

The Power of the Written Word

The simplest, most effective resilience technique to assist your mind and brain to manage the issues that life can present us with is to embrace the concept of writing things down. I use this technique regularly in my clinical work. When some issue is disturbing your emotional mind, your logical mind often struggles to become involved. This occurs because the emotional mind and brain are more powerful than the logical mind and brain. But when you write things down on paper, the more logical, rational parts of your brain are switched on, so you can examine the issue with greater clarity. This can be a powerful tool to reshape people's thinking and behaviour.

Countless people find that the act of putting down on paper, in their own handwriting, what is going on in their emotional mind is a game-changer. Sometimes you may not grasp just how irrational your thinking and behaviour can be until you write it down and then, in the cold light of day, rationally analyse what you discover through this process.

The left PFC is more associated with language and cold, hard analysis. We will be recruiting this part of your brain to assist you in analysing and in providing potential solutions to information surfacing from what you have written down.

If you can learn how to harness this power through this process, then the techniques necessary to become a real pragmatist become much easier tasks.

Pragmatism is a Skill

It is important to realize from the outset that pragmatism is a skill. A skill is the ability to master some area of expertise. Traditionally we associate skills with artisans such as carpenters or electricians. But all of us have an innate capacity to acquire skills in a multitude of areas. Before acquiring any skill, such as driving a car, cooking, dancing or learning the piano, it is necessary to progress through several stages.

1. The first stage involves learning or developing the skill. This may involve acquiring information and techniques from somebody skilled in the area. As this information is new and strange, it requires significant mental concentration to absorb. It can also feel awkward initially when putting it into action. Just think of the first few lessons with a driving instructor to visualize these feelings.

2. The second stage involves you practising the skill repeatedly till it becomes more familiar. You feel increasingly comfortable putting it into action.

3. The third stage is reached when application of the skill in everyday life becomes routine and automatic. You no longer consciously think about using this skill in practice. It is embedded in your unconscious mind. One more skill you have mastered!

We have already discussed in chapter one how you use your right PFC to focus and concentrate on learning a new skill and how this has a straight line to your amygdala, where you experience emotions. So a lot of brainpower and emotional energy is being used at the beginning. When we develop and practise the skill, however, within a few months the brain tends to shift responsibility for the skill to our calmer and more rational left PFC and other parts of the brain such as the basal ganglia. This is why you feel calm and comfortable with the skill and are able to carry it out automatically.

It is also exciting to realize that when you are learning and acquiring new skills, something amazing is occurring in your brain. You begin to increase the amount of myelin around the neuron tracts involved in this process. Myelin is important in speeding up and making these tracts in the brain more efficient. It makes your brain more efficient and effective. It also explains why the more often you practise the skill, the easier you will find it. You are literally rewiring your own brain!

When acquiring the skill of pragmatism, the process is similar. I will be assisting you to initially learn the technique. You may find yourself feeling anxious or frustrated when first trying to put this skill into practice, and this is both expected and normal. The next step involves practising the skill repeatedly in everyday life. The more you practise, the more automatic the skill will become. Finally, the skill becomes part of you. Neither you nor your brain have to consciously think about it. You just do it! And in the process, you transform your life.

How to Develop the Skill of Pragmatism

Pragmatism, as stated earlier, is a skill whereby you become adept at quickly analysing problematic situations with a view to finding and putting into practice the most effective solutions. This suggests that you become increasingly effective at finding the short cut to how best to deal with practical everyday difficulties.

I am now going to introduce you to my five-question pragmatic blueprint, which will form the basis of how you can tackle change of any form in your life. Learning the skill of how to apply the following five questions to any problematic situation or change that may occur in your life can be life-transforming: a true blueprint for life. These are the building blocks for making you more resilient in terms of how you cope with and adapt to periods of stressful change. If you can learn to apply this blueprint on a regular basis, you will notice how your capacity to cope with adversity will dramatically increase.

Think about a change you are currently experiencing in your life where you find yourself struggling. If nothing immediately comes to mind, think about the last time you experienced this scenario. Now, I want you to write down the details of this example into a notebook and then take a shot at trying to analyse the situation or issue you've chosen by answering the following five questions:

1. **How is this situation making me feel?** (Is it making you feel anxious or frustrated, for example?)
2. **What is it about this situation that is causing me to feel this way?**

3. **What in my thinking is preventing me from dealing with this situation?**
4. **What in my behaviour is preventing me from dealing with this situation?**
5. **How can I short-circuit these thinking and behavioural blocks to deal more effectively with this situation?**

How did you do? You probably found this exercise to be quite challenging to begin with and this is what I would expect, as it is unlikely that you have ever broken down such situations in this manner. Don't worry at this stage if you found yourself struggling. The rest of this book will assist you to learn how to apply this five-question resilience blueprint to any situation you will find yourself facing.

This process feels quite strange when you do it for the first time but, as with all skills, with time and practice you will become more comfortable applying this pragmatic blueprint. Nonetheless, immediately you might notice how you are already looking at the problematic situation in a completely different manner. This is because you are turning the full force of your rational brain towards analysing what it is about the change that is bothering you and, more importantly, what you can do to manage the situation differently. Be sure to keep your notebook with you as you read this book, as you will be applying this process regularly over the weeks and months to come.

Now let's try to unpack these five questions in more detail and show how they would work in practice by applying them to the following hypothetical example:

You have applied for a highly prized job at a major international company and have gone through a series of online, phone and face-to-face interviews. You are now one of two candidates remaining and you feel that you are best placed to get the post – you are even planning your new life in another country! It is so exciting. Then, instead of *that* phone call, you get an email letting you know that you have been unsuccessful. The new life you had built up around the post disappears in an instant. Within a few days, you become emotionally depressed, withdraw socially from friends and family, drink excessively and ruminate constantly about the situation.

If you applied our blueprint, the answers might look like this:

1. **How is this situation making me feel? (Is it making you feel anxious or frustrated, for example?)**
   The answer here is quite simple: 'I am feeling emotionally depressed.'

2. **What is it about this situation that is causing me to feel this way?**
   This question is based on the concept that, in life, it is not what happens to us that makes us feel emotionally distressed, but instead how we are looking at or interpreting it. In other words, it is how are you thinking about the situation which is making you distressed. Why is the situation bothering you at all? In this case, you are asking yourself: what is it about missing out on this post that is causing me to feel depressed?
   The answer here might be: 'I am feeling depressed because I believe that I was not good enough in the eyes of the recruiters. I failed in my task of getting the job, and because of this, I believe that I am a failure.'

3. **What in my thinking is preventing me from dealing with this situation?**

This question is based on the concept that most of us develop fixed ways of thinking about situations, which are often irrational and unhelpful and prevent us from dealing with the situation. In this example, the answer might be: 'It is my fixed belief that because I failed this job interview, I am a failure as a person.'

4.   **What in my behaviour is preventing me from dealing with this situation?**

This question is based on the concept that how we behave as a result of our emotional reaction to a situation can either hinder or help us deal with it. Unfortunately, much of the time our behavioural responses only worsen the situation and delay or prevent us from dealing with it.

In this example the answer might be: 'It is my ruminating, social withdrawal, refusal to look at other options and excessive drinking as a consequence of feeling emotionally depressed which are blocking me from managing the situation.'

5.   **How can I short-circuit these thinking and behavioural blocks to deal more effectively with this situation?**

This assumes that you have already explored your emotional, thinking and behavioural responses to the situation through the previous four questions. It then challenges you to see how you could bypass any unhelpful thinking patterns or negative behaviours to deal with the situation more effectively.

In this example, it is clear that the major thinking block is your belief that 'I as a person can be classified as a failure simply because I was unsuccessful at a job application'. This of course makes no sense. The more pragmatic approach would be to accept that human beings cannot be classified as either a success or a failure as a person but can obviously be successful or fail at a task such as a job application. That sort of failure is a part of life and one of the ways in which we learn. The only real failure is not getting back up again, so you might need to go through a number of similar applications before you land the job of your dreams.

The negative behavioural blocks in this example that you have to tackle are pretty obvious. 'I will have to reduce my alcohol intake, share how I feel with my friends and family and seek out new job opportunities for the future.'

Before moving on to a real-life case study, it is worth noting that to become truly pragmatic and resilient, it is really helpful to reflect on and absorb some of the following ten insights, many of which will be explored throughout this book:

1. The importance of unconditional self-acceptance, where we accept ourselves for the wonderful, unique, special human beings that each of us are but also accept responsibility for our behaviours or actions.
2. Life is often unfair and discomfort is a part of life.
3. The world is an uncertain place, over which we have little or no control.
4. Failure is an innate part of life and the means by which we develop and grow as human beings, and the only failure in life is not getting back up and trying again.
5. There is never a perfect solution to the difficulties and woes of life, just the best solution we can come up with at that moment in time.

6. Catastrophizing about how awful things could be is a waste of our valuable time and energies, which are best spent on more productive matters.

7. Life in general is too short to waste time on unnecessary trivial conflicts and arguments. Remember: if you don't get into the ring, you cannot have a fight.

8. If you can learn to stop taking yourself too seriously and develop a sense of humour about yourself and life, it becomes easier to deal with what life throws at you.

9. Procrastination or delaying tasks due to anxiety or frustration will only paralyse your capacity to cope with change. Learning how to problem-solve and deal more efficiently with such tasks will bear much fruit.

10. Improving your empathy skills, where you learn how to see into the hearts and minds of another human being, will greatly assist you in dealing with the many difficulties that life can generate.

It might be useful to write down these ten insights in your notebook and keep referring back to them when applying our five-question blueprint to your life. You will see them being applied in practice when dealing with the different life situations described later in the book. If you can absorb some of these messages or insights, then applying the blueprint becomes an easier task to achieve.

Tom's Story

Tom, out of the blue, is asked by his boss to take over a new project but finds himself becoming rapidly overwhelmed. He becomes extremely anxious, almost panicky. He feels out of his depth as this new project is going to require some 'out of the box' thinking, which he has never been especially good at doing. He begins to catastrophize as to the awful mess he will make of the task and how much of a failure he will be when this happens. He procrastinates for weeks, constantly delaying getting stuck in to the task, which allows the 'monster in his mind' to enlarge further. To make matters worse, Tom is also a perfectionist. Unless he can complete any task perfectly, he struggles to perform it at all. Matters get worse when his boss informs him that he is hopeful that Tom will be ready to present his plans to a group of his peers in a month's time. No pressure!

If Tom was applying our blueprint, it would look like this:

1. **How is this situation making me feel?**
   'My overwhelming emotions are anxiety and panic. I am also feeling slightly ashamed.'
2. **What is it about this situation that is causing me to feel this way?**
   'I am feeling anxious, mainly because I am unsure as to how well-equipped I am to carry out this task, and am only able to visualize the mess that I am going to make of it. I am also anxious as I know if I cannot do a good job here that I would be a failure to myself and others.

I am feeling embarrassed or ashamed as I know that my colleagues will see that I am not as good at my job as they would expect.'

3. **What in my thinking is preventing me from dealing with this situation?**

    'I have convinced myself that I am not good enough to do it and unable to think outside the box. I am a perfectionist, so cannot cope with the thought that my final result would not be perfect. I am spending too much time concentrating on what might go wrong and not enough on how to sort out the problem. I am also falling into the trap of both rating or judging myself as a failure and allowing others to do likewise, instead of accepting that the only thing I should be rating is how effectively I manage to carry out this task.'

4. **What in my behaviour is preventing me from dealing with this situation?**

    'It is pretty obvious what I am doing wrong in relation to my behaviour. I am delaying, delaying and delaying getting stuck into the job I have been asked to do. I am also "playing my boss along" by reassuring him that all is well, which is only adding to the pressure I am feeling. I am also looking at the task as a whole, and as a result am feeling overwhelmed.'

5. **How can I short-circuit my thinking and behavioural blocks to deal more effectively with this situation?**

    'If I am going to resolve this crisis, I am going to have to change how I am thinking about the task and also my behaviour.

    'In relation to my "thinking", I am going to have to accept that this is a new challenge for me and approach it as an opportunity to learn, rather than a potential disaster. I need to stop looking at what might go wrong and focus on getting the job done instead. I have to put my desire for perfectionism to one side here and focus on simply getting the job done to the best of my ability. I have to cease believing that I can be rated as a person by myself or others, but accept that the results of my project can be rated. But if I have done my best, I am off the hook.

'In relation to my "behaviour", I need to "get off my butt" and get stuck in to doing this project as I was asked to do. If I am struggling with some new concepts or ideas, I need to research potential solutions or seek advice from colleagues or peers as to how to manage them. I could also decide to break the project up into smaller chunks, which might make it seem less overwhelming. I could then begin to tackle these smaller sections day by day and week by week, making sure that the final product was ready a few days before my presentation so that I could edit it appropriately.

'Perhaps it might also be wiser to own up to my boss if I am really struggling with areas of the project and seek out further advice from either him or colleagues he might assign to assist me.'

The good news is that Tom, as a result of adapting the above approach, does manage to produce a decent project plan, which goes down well with his boss and colleagues. He does have to call in some assistance from his boss, who notes that he was surprised that Tom had not come to him sooner as he was aware this was a difficult and challenging project. He assigns a junior assistant to help him with the necessary research. Tom also learns how to break up the project into chunks and, with the assistance of his new helper, begins to rapidly sort out the nuts and bolts of the project. In the process of delivering the project through an application of the above pragmatic approaches, Tom learns much about himself and how to handle future stressful situations, which he hopes to apply from now on. In practice, however, Tom will have to apply the above pragmatic approach to many similar situations over the following three to six months if he wishes to become truly adept at applying the skill of pragmatism!

Pragmatism and Change

Now that we have explored the skill of pragmatism and how you too can develop and learn the appropriate techniques, let's turn our attention to how you can apply this skill to managing periods of significant change in your life.

At the heart of all change lies the world of problem-solving. Even if the cause of change is a joyous one, such as the arrival of a new baby into your house, there are still a series of practical problems to be resolved, as any new parent will attest. When the cause of the change in question is more negative, such as the arrival of a sudden illness affecting a loved one, for example a major heart attack or cancer, matters can become more challenging. In such situations, what is creating your distress is usually the arrival of a new set of problems or difficulties which were not present beforehand. These may threaten on occasion to overwhelm you emotionally.

This is where pragmatism reigns supreme. It provides a simple blueprint for handling such difficult periods in your life. It allows you to quickly and efficiently explore how such periods are affecting you emotionally, the thinking and behavioural blocks which are obstructing you to move forward, and enables you to lay out a platform as to how best to deal with these blocks and problem-solve the issues in question.

This is the blueprint that we will use for the remainder of this book. We will first identify the principal emotions that such periods of change are engendering in us. This will act as a signpost to the most likely thinking and behavioural blocks that are obstructing us in dealing with such periods. This enables us to then lay out some practical solutions to problem-solve these blocks, allowing us to deal quickly and effectively with the issues involved.

I have discovered over decades of working with people struggling with change that there are seven common emotions which are most triggered at such times. These are:

1. Anxiety
2. Frustration
3. Depression
4. Hurt
5. Shame
6. Sadness
7. Regret

Underlying each one of these emotions are different thinking and behavioural blocks that prevent us from handling change effectively. As we have already covered, age is irrelevant here as we are inclined to think and act in a similar manner, often independent of it. It is more about the belief systems that each of us have developed as a consequence of our childhood, adolescence, young adulthood or adult experiences. We have already noted how, when Tom was able to name his emotions and from there identify the thinking and behavioural blocks which were obstructing him deal with his project, he was able to sort the issues out. It will be important for you, too, to constantly refer back to your notebook, detailing your emotional menu, if you are unsure of which feelings are being triggered by a particular change in your life circumstances. It might also assist you, when using this book, to go to the chapter of relevance to the emotion in question. This is perfectly fine, but I would strongly counsel returning to read the other chapters as well, as each will equip you with skills you may need for the future.

One final yet important caveat to the approach we will be using. We will be discussing a wide variety of situations and issues in the pages which follow. There will be many situations where you may find the assistance of a therapist, doctor or specialist extremely valuable in dealing with these issues, and if so, please use this facility. This can be especially the case if the situation in question is complex or emotionally distressing. Some may also find it difficult to apply these concepts without the assistance of a therapist. Others may prefer a completely different therapeutic approach from the one presented, and that too is absolutely fine. Each person must find their own road when it comes to managing change in their lives. It has been my experience, however, that those who practise the above pragmatic approach and apply it regularly to their lives often describe it as life-altering. If you are still interested, read on.

PART TWO

ANXIETY

3. Why Change Can Make You Anxious

Significant swathes of the population find change usually makes them feel anxious, even on occasion panicky. You may notice this emotion in yourself as a natural response to some significant change in your life. It may be that you suddenly lose your job, a family member or close friend becomes ill, a relationship breaks down. There are so many upheavals in life that can throw us into a spin and neither you nor I can dodge these times. They are a part of life.

As already discussed, your emotional reactions to any negative event will depend on how you think about it, which in turn depends on whether the event triggers your irrational beliefs or not. Similarly, your behavioural responses will also depend on the emotions triggered. So it is with anxiety.

The good news is that there are some well-trodden thinking and behavioural paths that those who respond to change with anxiety tend to travel, and this allows us to explore the ways in which anxiety shows up in your thinking. More importantly, it opens up some new and exciting pragmatic approaches to prevent yourself travelling down such paths in the future. A life-changing possibility. Let's explore some of these pitfalls in greater detail.

Uncertainty

As human beings, many of us tend to become extremely anxious, even panicky, when faced with absolute uncertainty – where you can no longer control the outcome of a situation and all your previously assumed certainties seem to have been blown out of the water.

There are reasons why the last sudden economic crash triggered such an epidemic of anxiety in many countries. Suddenly it dawned on us, as individuals and communities, that none of us are truly in control of what happens, despite what we think. The spectre of uncertainty entered our lives. Solid foundations turned out to be shifting sands. You cannot be certain, for example, whether the job you occupy at this moment in time may suddenly be gone, depending on economic circumstances or the vagaries of large multinational companies. Or whether an accident or illness might suddenly enter your life, creating financial instability for you and your loved ones.

Such changes in our economic circumstances can present us with the ultimate uncertainty challenge, with no definite answers as to how matters will pan out. If your natural response to significant changes such as this or of the type detailed in the previous chapter is to demand 100 per cent or absolute certainty as to the outcome, you are going to find yourself struggling with anxiety.

This demand often emanates from the irrational belief systems discussed in chapter two. It may be, for example, that you grew up in a household where being in control was a mantra and any concept of uncertainty barely tolerated. Later we will meet people struggling with this demand and see how they used pragmatism to overcome it.

The reason why we struggle with uncertainty is that we tend to surround ourselves with routines and structures in our simple everyday lives which reassure us incorrectly that we are 'in control'. I owe much to my colleague, leading CBT therapist and trainer Enda Murphy (www.seeme.ie), for his insights into this concept. Because we find ourselves generally 'winning' in these areas, we deceive ourselves into believing that this is the way life is and should be. We know what time we will get up, what we will have for breakfast, which social media and news feeds we will follow, what we will have for lunch, which films or Netflix series we will watch and so on.

But is there actually anything (apart from death and taxes, of course) that you can be 100 per cent or absolutely certain about? The answer is, of course, no. Life has at its core a deep-rooted uncertainty.

It is interesting to note that the 'Uncertainty Principle' even underlies the world of quantum mechanics, seen as the basis of modern science, with the greatest scientific and mathematical minds still struggling with the concept of uncertainty up to the present moment. The underlying reason for this struggle is that the laws of mathematics break down when one moves into the subatomic or quantum world. Science doesn't like uncertainty, even at a quantum level. Yet, despite this uncertainty, scientists have learned to live with it. And if they have, so must we!

None of us can know from minute to minute or hour to hour what life can suddenly throw at us. The best we can hope for in life is reasonable certainty and even this can be quickly blown away by events. So, what can you do?

The pragmatic approach to uncertainty accepts that in life there is always a percentage chance that something will or won't happen and that we must learn to accept this reality and build it into our lives. The percentage risk may be, and often is, extremely small, but it is still always there. In this scenario, the belief that our everyday lives are under our control is therefore a mirage. It might only take a phone call from the hospital as you are going out the door with your partner for a night out, to say that your mother has had a stroke, to blow away such 'certainties'! In one of my previous books, *Emotional Resilience*, I recommend the 'Coin Exercise' for those who continue to struggle with this reality and refer you to this for further information. Here, however, we will be demonstrating later how to apply such pragmatic insights into common situations which are making us anxious.

Catastrophizing

Another reason why change makes us anxious is that it triggers a deep-seated evolutionary tendency to catastrophize, or visualize the 'worst-case scenario'. It is the right PFC that controls this tendency to catastrophize. In the past this was a really useful skill for human beings, as it allowed us to dodge potentially dangerous situations. We could map out potential trails through 'enemy country', for example, and visualize which ones might present the greatest risk to our survival and, by avoiding them, stay safe and well. Most of us have found our right PFC to be in overdrive when faced with situations that trigger our anxiety. A good example is health phobias, where we regularly find ourselves visualizing arriving in hospital acutely ill or at risk of dying, with no actual evidence of an underlying serious medical condition.

Whilst this function of the PFC in certain situations (such as finding ourselves inadvertently in an area of the city which is prone to muggings) can be useful, for some of us, visualizing danger or catastrophizing can develop a life of its own. We see 'danger' in everything around us, even when such risks are extremely small.

If change is making you extremely anxious, there is a good chance that you are catastrophizing wildly. There may only be a tiny per-cent chance that something might go awry, but you are focusing primarily on this percentage. Your best friend is suddenly admitted to hospital with chest pain, for example, and by the end of the day you are already planning her funeral and wondering how you are going to cope with her loss! The reality being that she is in hospital simply for tests to rule out any underlying major health issues such as heart disease.

One of the more distressing aspects of catastrophizing is its tendency, within our emotional mind, to cascade. This is where one false catastrophic assumption rapidly leads to the next, and so on. In the above example, you may notice how you allowed your emotional mind to move from the situation where you hear your best friend is in hospital with chest pain, to deciding she is going to die, to her death, to planning her funeral! Because your emotional mind is stronger than your rational mind, the former – if allowed – can run riot. Change presents the right PFC and your emotional mind with rich material for this to happen.

The pragmatic approach to catastrophizing would involve accepting that almost 90 per cent of what we worry about never happens. You are simply using up unnecessary time and energy that could be better employed in more sensible pursuits, such as looking after the physical and mental wellbeing of yourself, partner and family, in that order. Often when such catastrophic thoughts are committed to paper, our rational mind can begin to see them for what they are and dismiss them. We will see this in practice later.

Struggling to Cope

Another reason you may become anxious as a consequence of some significant period of change is that you believe you will simply not cope. You may, for example, irrationally believe that if what you are catastrophizing about were to happen, you will be completely unable to cope with the consequences. Suppose you have experienced a major long-term relationship break-up and are catastrophizing that you are going to finish up alone and lonely. Your emotional mind may then try to convince you that you will be completely unable to cope if this happens. The more you reflect on this reality, the stronger this belief can become, till being unable to cope is all that you can see.

The pragmatic approach to this false belief would present you with the blunt question – 'If what you are catastrophizing happens, are you going to simply sit down in the middle of the floor, throw your hands to the heavens and decide that it is all over and that you can't progress any further?' The answer is, of course, no! The reality is that no matter what happens to you, however significant or emotionally distressing the change is, you will inexorably and inevitably move forward. You will simply not have the luxury of 'giving up'. You will still wake up in the morning, have a shower, get dressed and continue the normal routines of life, work, shopping, coping with family issues and so on.

Why do we cope? We cope because it is in our own interests and in the interests of those we love. Try to explain to a small child that you are giving up, when a loved partner dies tragically and your whole world is crumbling around you. Clearly, in such awful circumstances, you will still have to feed, dress and love the little one. You do not have the luxury of 'not coping'. It will be your inner reserves, and their love, that will hopefully assist you to survive such a nightmare scenario.

Self-rating

Another common reason why change makes us anxious is that it is commonly associated with self-judgement or self-rating. This is where you allow your emotional mind to berate you, sometimes mercilessly, if you cannot achieve the impossible demands that you may be making on yourself.

Let's take a simple example where change has turned your life upside down. Your company decides that they are putting you on shorter working hours, due to financial constraints. You are struggling emotionally and practically to come to terms with your new situation. In a WhatsApp chat with some colleagues, many of them seem to be coping admirably with their new situation. You find yourself becoming increasingly anxious and stressed. 'What am "I" doing wrong? Why are they coping so well while I struggle? I am such a failure!'

Here, you are allowing your emotional mind to berate you, the person, as a failure, if you are unable to cope with your new situation as well as your work colleagues seem to be doing.

The pragmatic approach to rating is to challenge whether a human being can be rated at all. Each of us is special and unique, and so the only things you can rate in life are your behaviours and actions, including skills and hobbies. In the situation above, you would have to be kind to yourself, accept that you are coping as well as you can in difficult circumstances, and move on.

The Role of Your Behaviour

Now that we've looked at the ways in which anxiety can affect how we think about change, it's important to consider how anxiety affects our behaviour. Because how you respond behaviourally when change makes you anxious can sometimes add to the problem. Let's explore three common behaviours and see how a more pragmatic approach might assist you.

Avoidant Behaviour

One response to becoming anxious about some significant change is to avoid dealing with it. A simple example might be where you are suddenly promoted at work but fail to tell your boss and colleagues about having significant social anxiety about work presentations. Instead of trying to deal with the issue, you keep avoiding such presentations, coming up with multiple excuses to pass the task on to other colleagues.

Avoidance when faced with some significant change such as this will just make you feel increasingly stressed and anxious. Other examples, such as avoiding opening up letters from the bank or possible bills if you are faced with sudden changes in financial circumstances, or avoiding other people if you are diagnosed with a bout of depression, will also make your anxiety levels soar.

The pragmatic approach would challenge whether avoiding dealing with the causes or consequences of change is assisting you to confront the issue. It would then encourage you to ditch the avoidance and get on with dealing with the change that is causing you to feel anxious to begin with.

Safety Behaviour

Another common response if you are anxious in change situations is to apply safety behaviour to try to reduce your anxiety. Let's suppose that you have suddenly developed a motorway phobia and this change is making you increasingly anxious. You could of course use avoidant behaviour. But you can also attempt some safety behaviours or techniques such as travelling the back roads instead 'for safety' or ensuring there is always someone else in the car with you if having to take the motorway.

The purpose of your safety behaviour is, of course, to make you feel less anxious. Unfortunately, it may end with you feeling even more anxious the next time you have to take the motorway!

The pragmatic approach would challenge whether applying such safety behaviours was helping or hindering you from dealing with the issue, the latter being more likely, and would encourage you to cease them.

Procrastinating Behaviour

A final unhealthy behaviour when dealing with change is procrastination. Where you keep putting off 'getting into the ring' with the difficulties that change can present. You will usually find yourself procrastinating due to some of the reasons mentioned above – uncertainty, catastrophizing, fear that you will be unable to cope, or believing that you are a failure. The longer you procrastinate, the longer it will take to resolve the matter in question.

Maybe you are someone who keeps putting off tasks at work. You are suddenly presented with an unusual one and become increasingly anxious. Maybe you will mess it up or miss out on some crucial data? It could turn out to be a disaster and how would you cope? The best thing is therefore to keep putting off the task, as this makes you feel less anxious. Alas, the time for completion is nearing!

The pragmatic approach to procrastination would challenge whether such delaying behaviours are assisting you in dealing with the cause of your distress, namely an unusual task. It would encourage you to break the task up into chunks and a timeline and problem-solve each section. Before you know it, the task will be done and your anxiety levels a lot lower!

4. How to Manage Your 'Change' Anxiety

In the previous chapter, we explored how change can make you anxious and how your behaviours can add to this. Now let's see if pragmatism could assist you to overcome these obstacles and, in the process, diminish or banish your change-driven anxiety.

The Pragmatic Approach to Change-driven Anxiety

In chapter two, we drew up a blueprint that involved answering five pragmatic questions to assist you in managing any significant change in your life. Let's now apply this blueprint to Jason, who is experiencing one of the commonest causes of change-driven anxiety amongst our young student population, namely taking the wrong course at college.

Choosing a Higher Education Course
It is difficult, some would say impossible, for a young person in their late teens to know for certain which Higher Education course is best suited to them, or indeed what they really want to do with their lives. They are asked in their final years of school, while they are still quite young and under pressure to do well in

exams, to make such choices. Inevitably, many find themselves on the wrong course and stumped. This can lead to periods of great stress and anxiety. It is hard enough to cope with the huge changes associated with leaving home or school to enter the larger landscape of college, without having to face the truth that the course chosen may be the wrong one! This is what happens to Jason. Let's see how he uses our pragmatic blueprint to manage his anxiety levels, when faced with such a period of change.

Jason's Story

Jason is a nineteen-year-old student who realizes halfway through his first year at college that he is in trouble. He has never been absolutely sure as to which course to take, so he decided to apply for an engineering degree, as he enjoyed maths at school. Within months of starting the course, he is struggling, increasingly realizing that he feels like a square peg in a round hole. Apart from the normal difficulties of coming to terms with college itself, as he is from a rural background, he now realizes to his horror that he simply hates the course and that he has made a big mistake. On chatting to others, it is increasingly clear that computer science would have been a better bet. He now feels trapped, unsure of what to do.

His anxiety levels begin to soar. The more anxious he becomes, the more physical symptoms he develops, including tension headaches, his stomach permanently in knots, struggling to sleep and finding it difficult to concentrate on anything. Jason knows that he should make his parents and college authorities aware of his difficulties but, as is his wont, he procrastinates. His assignments suffer and this makes him increasingly anxious. He compensates by using alcohol in copious amounts to dampen his anxiety. He begins to feel a little flat in mood and even skips some lectures. How can he get out of the mess he has created for himself? He shares his woes with a college friend who encourages him to chat to the on-campus counsellor. This proves to be a turning point. She encourages him to use a pragmatic approach, which involves answering five key questions on paper, to analyse his current situation. Jason finds this approach extremely effective.

Here are Jason's findings:

1. **How does this situation make me feel?**
   'My main emotion is anxiety.'
2. **What is it about this situation that is causing me to feel this way?**
   'I am feeling anxious as I'm completely unsure or uncertain as to how this situation is going to pan out. If I tell my parents, will they be very annoyed and feel that I have let them down? If I tell the college authorities, will they prevent me from changing to a different course? But I am most anxious that a move to computer science might also fail to work out. I know it is going to be awful, no matter which way I look at this. I have always wanted to come to college and now I am wasting my chance. If I stay on the course, I will feel miserable, and if I change to a different course, it may be the wrong choice. I have to be sure if I change that it works out. If not, I am a failure.'

3. **What in my thinking is preventing me from dealing with this situation?**

   'I am demanding that the next course I choose must be the right one, and that my parents and the college must assist me to make this happen. I am also visualizing the worst-case scenario even though nothing has technically happened to date. I haven't even spoken to either my parents or the college authorities about this matter, but already assume this will turn out badly.'

4. **What in my behaviour is preventing me from dealing with this situation?**

   'I am putting my head in the sand and hoping that it will all go away without actually doing something to change my situation. I am creating difficulties for myself by not engaging with my parents and the college. It is also pretty clear that the drinking and dodging lectures is not helping my case.'

5. **How can I short-circuit my thinking and behavioural blocks to deal more effectively with this situation?**

   'In relation to my flawed thinking, I need to accept some harsh realities. It is difficult at the age of eighteen to choose the right college course, so I have to accept this and be kinder to myself. There are also no absolute certainties that any course I do choose will be the right one. Perhaps some intensive research, however, might improve my chances of picking the best one. There is also little point in spending my time and especially my energies in visualizing just how awful things might get. The reality is that, with luck, none of the negative outcomes that I am catastrophizing about will ever happen.

My parents love me and I am sure they will help, and the college authorities are also there to assist students who are struggling. Unless either of these situations change, I am better off putting my energies into solving the problem.

'In relation to my behaviour, it's time to take my head out of the sand and contact my parents and the college, to see about leaving this course and moving sideways. I also need to stop my alcohol binges and focus instead on doing further research into computer science and related subjects, to see if they seem more suitable.'

The good news is that by applying the above approaches and with the assistance of his college counsellor Jason finds it easier to manage this extremely challenging period of change in his life. He has an emotional chat with his parents, who are very supportive. The college authorities are also extremely helpful and lay out some options for him, such as finishing his current year and then switching over to another course. He decides to do this, and the following year finds himself on a computer course, which he has researched properly before making the jump. He takes to it like a duck to water. Moreover, he has now developed a new pragmatic approach to solve similar life issues which will occur in the future. As he admits to his counsellor, perhaps this skill will be more relevant than anything he learns in college, the capacity to adapt and think outside the box.

Let's now meet Ellen, Joe and Maeve, each of them struggling with a particular transitional period of problematic change in their lives. They, too, find the above pragmatic approach immensely helpful in resolving their difficulties. You may even see yourself in some of these cases!

The Menopause

Let's begin by meeting Ellen. She is encountering a period of change in her life; a phase that can be so problematic for many women, namely the menopause. This menopause normally arrives somewhere between forty-five and fifty-five years of age, when the ovaries begin to shut down production of the female hormone oestrogen. This can lead to the sudden arrival of a host of physical and psychological changes with which many women struggle to cope.

Lots of women will relate to Ellen's story and her coming to terms with what is a very challenging phase for them.

Ellen's Story

Ellen is forty-eight years old and happily married to Peter; they have two children. She works as a legal secretary and is just beginning to enjoy her newfound freedom as her two children have left for college. She has noticed over the previous two years how her periods were becoming more infrequent and of shorter duration. She assumes that she is just coming up to 'that time', as other friends called the menopause. But nothing really prepares her for the changes coming her way.

Suddenly her periods stop completely. Over the months that follow she develops dreadful sweats and flushes, especially at night, when sleep becomes impossible. She throws off sheets and blankets and even considers moving to a different bedroom as she is constantly waking Peter up. She also notices a deterioration in her skin and hair quality.

Then there is the extreme dryness in the vaginal area, which makes intimacy with Peter increasingly uncomfortable. She finds herself making excuses to avoid sex, which creates difficulties in their relationship.

Cognitively she finds herself slowing down and becoming more forgetful. One day, for example, whilst doing a series of tasks around the town, she returns home with some grocery shopping to find that she has already bought the same items earlier. It takes Peter most of the evening to calm her down, reassuring her that she is not developing dementia. She finds herself becoming embarrassed when flushes suddenly appear when chatting to friends or colleagues, making her increasingly anxious that this might happen again.

But the psychological effects of these changes surprise her most. Ellen finds herself becoming increasingly anxious and occasionally finds her mood dropping for short periods. She struggles with the uncertainty created by these changes and what they would mean for her and Peter moving forward in their lives. She also worries that she will be unable to cope if the symptoms deteriorate. Her greatest battle, however, is with herself, as she increasingly sees herself as 'lesser', 'worthless' and now different or 'abnormal' in comparison with her previous life.

Ellen also finds herself catastrophizing. She begins to believe that she is 'less of a woman' as a result of the physical changes noted above, that she is less attractive to Peter and to others, and that the most important part of her life is over. She also becomes increasingly anxious that she will never be able to sleep properly at night due to the sweats.

Her lack of sleep leads Ellen to become increasingly irritable with her husband, children and work colleagues.

This is foreign to her as she is normally a sunny person. After six months, her previously wonderful life and world has been turned upside down.

Ellen discusses matters with close female friends and her sister, some of whom are at different stages of this process. They have all tried to handle the menopause in varied ways, and she finds herself increasingly confused. Her sister suggests that she chats to her GP and considers hormone replacement therapy (HRT). Ellen is horrified at this prospect as she has heard some nightmare stories about the latter; how it piles on weight and, according her trusted friend Dr Google, is associated with increased risks of breast cancer and heart disease. She is also falling under the spell of social media, where she despairs on observing how other women seem to be coping so well with this phase. This made her increasingly anxious as she can see no way out of her current dilemma. The more anxious she becomes, the greater her fatigue, and she is now wracked with tension headaches and irritable bowel symptoms. As she confides to a close friend, her life is slowly descending into a nightmare.

What is really happening to Ellen is that apart from the real, unpleasant and uncomfortable physical symptoms which the withdrawal of oestrogen is producing in her body, the hormonal changes are upsetting her emotional brain. She is struggling with uncertainty, catastrophizing and self-rating. This is being worsened by her lack of sleep. Her behaviour is also not helping. She is procrastinating about going to see her family doctor for some professional advice, choosing instead to take advice from Dr Google, the most anxiety-causing information source of all! Her social-media world, where she seeks solace, only succeeds in making her more anxious, creating a false image of what the menopause is really like for the vast majority of women.

Let's see what happens when Ellen chooses instead to apply our pragmatic blueprint and to answer the five questions it contains.

Here is Ellen's blueprint:

1. **How is this situation making me feel?**
   'The menopause is making me feel emotionally and physically anxious.'

2. **What is it about this situation that is causing me to feel this way?**
   'I am feeling anxious and totally unsure of how long this awful phase of my life will continue. How will it affect my relationship? How long will these flushes and sweats last? Am I going to be seen as less attractive by Peter? Will the difficulties with intimacy destroy our relationship? Are my difficulties with memory and concentration going to get worse? Where is all this going?

   'I know I am only looking at the negative side here. I can only see a future dominated by flushes, sweats, sleep and memory difficulties and a permanent battle with skin, hair and vaginal dryness. Not to mention on bad days, the thought that Peter might leave, unable to cope with me any longer!

   'I know that I am beating myself up as a result of these changes, considering myself as ugly and lesser, and also anxious that other friends and colleagues might observe my flushes.'

3. **What in my thinking is preventing me from dealing with this situation?**

'I am demanding absolute certainty that all of these physical and emotional symptoms will settle down quickly. I am also catastrophizing about the possible scenarios which could happen due to this sudden change in my life, such as Peter leaving me, for example, even though I have no evidence that this will be the case. I am also self-rating myself as worthless, ugly and weird as a result of the menopause.'

4. **What in my behaviour is preventing me from dealing with this situation?**

'I am refusing to accept that I cannot handle this situation on my own and require professional assistance as my sister suggested. I am driving myself nuts by constantly seeking out information from Dr Google, much of which I do not understand and cannot apply to my specific situation. I am also believing false messages from Instagram and other sites, suggesting that other women in my situation are coping better with this period. Believing that if they are continuing to keep themselves looking so attractive and competent, there must be something wrong with me.'

5. **How can I short-circuit my thinking and behavioural blocks to deal more effectively with this situation?**

'In relation to my flawed thinking, I am going to have to accept that the menopause is a natural, if extremely unpleasant, experience for many women and that I am no different. It would also be more useful to acquire some proper information about how long it will last and how best to manage it, rather than remaining constantly anxious about being unable to control what is going to happen in the future.

'I will also have to stop visualizing the worst-case scenarios which might occur due to the menopause and focus instead on problem-solving the different physical and emotional issues that it presents. I will cope. I have coped with the task of delivering and rearing two lovely children. This is just a new suite of issues to be faced down. I was never one to step away from a challenge in my life and I will face this one down too.

'Above all, I need to be kinder to myself and cease rating myself as lesser or ugly or worthless. What do these terms really mean when examined in the cold light of day? Am I not a special person who is much loved by Peter and my two children? This change in my life, even if unpleasant and completely unwished-for, does not define who I am. Rather, it is how I choose to deal with it that will define me in terms of my behaviour.

'In relation to my behaviour, it is high time I stop trying to deal with this unwanted change in my life on my own and seek out professional advice and assistance. It might be helpful to attend a female GP with whom I would be comfortable when sharing my current dilemma. I require assistance and advice in relation to the sweats, flushes, vaginal dryness and intimacy, not to mention some reassurance that I am not developing dementia!

'I may have to listen to the doctor's suggestions, even if these include some short-term medications or other therapies to make this period more tolerable. I am also determined to switch off Dr Google as it is only making me increasingly anxious and despairing. Maybe it is also time to delete some social-media apps and confide instead in more face-to-face conversations with people I trust.'

Let's now discover what happens when Ellen decides, following this pragmatic analysis of the arrival of the menopause into her life, to put these decisions into action.

She firstly visits Dr Jill, revealing, with a few tears, how traumatic the previous six months have been and the physical and emotional torments she has endured. It turns out to be one of the most important discussions of her life to date. Ellen learns just what the menopause is. Where the sweats, flushes, dryness and sleep problems emanated from and the importance of her sex-hormone oestrogen. Why the ovaries cease to produce it and the consequences of this. How this period of change is usually time-lined, in terms of duration. How some of these changes will be permanent and the importance of developing good practical techniques to deal with them. The need to introduce sensible lifestyle changes, including diet, exercise, good sleep hygiene and reducing alcohol levels. How many of the emotional changes she is noticing, especially anxiety, are worsened by her shortage of oestrogen and resulting lack of sleep.

They have a frank conversation about the short-term use of oestrogen replacements, to tide her over the first year or so, in terms of sweats, flushes and sleep. Dr Jill explains the current guidelines as to their usage and how previous concerns about the use of HRT have been partially allayed, especially if used for shorter periods. The use of local vaginal therapies to assist with intimacy is also discussed. How it also takes time for the brain to adjust cognitively to the lack of oestrogen but how this gradually returns to normal. Above all, how most women struggle through the same set of physical and emotional consequences as Ellen, just maybe hiding them better. This makes Ellen feel better about herself and how she is coping. She now has a better understanding of the menopause and how to manage it.

She puts all of this advice into action. The lifestyle changes and HRT transform her life. Her sweats and flushes greatly diminish. Her sleep improves, as does her relationship with Peter, following an emotional discussion where she reveals what had been going on in great detail, together with the usage of suitable local preparations. Her confidence slowly but surely returns. She has permanently ditched her social-media apps and is finding one-to-one conversations with friends more nourishing. She accepts that she is never going to return to her pre-menopausal state but has now learned pragmatically how to adjust and cope with her new changed state.

The Covid-19 Pandemic

Let's now meet Joe and his encounter with one of the most significant periods of change since the last world war, namely the Covid-19 pandemic. It is unsurprising that anxiety has been the overwhelming emotional response to the changes this virus has forced upon our everyday lives. This is understandable as it – like all pandemics – has blown away much of what we believed to be certain. So often in life you can find yourself worrying and anxious about what might happen in the future, without much basis for your worries. Covid-19, however, gave us all something solid to be anxious about, in relation to the health of ourselves and loved ones, and our economic and financial security going forward. Everything seemed suddenly fluid and uncertain.

We had the sudden emergence of a virus that swept into our midst, incredibly infectious and seemingly random in nature; some people ended up in intensive care and on ventilators, while others had a benign course. It was a virus that seemed destined to come in waves, the timing of which was often uncertain and random. It was a fickle organism, often affecting men more than women, mainly bypassing small children, while ravaging those over the ages of seventy-five to eighty.

Most countries and continents have been devastated by the virus's effects, with only a few escaping with less illness and death. Countless people have died and many have been left with post-viral complications. Fear as to how this virus might affect ourselves and our loved ones has been endemic in almost every country. The Covid-19 pandemic, like its predecessors, swept across our planet, leaving all of us fearful and apprehensive about the future. As with most pandemics, vaccination presents the best chance of dealing with this one. Uncertainty still exists, however, as to when our lives can fully return to normal.

We will explore in chapter seventeen the world of grief and how distressing it can be to lose a partner, parent, child, sibling or close friend. This distress has been compounded by restrictions imposed to combat this virus, which has made it even more difficult to mourn the passing of loved ones.

There have also been significant social and mental-health effects involved in locking down whole countries or communities whilst this pandemic raged. The virus uprooted everything which we felt to be secure and certain. Suddenly we could no longer hug each other or bury our dead with dignity, and were required to treat each other like pariahs rather than fellow human beings, wear masks and constantly wash our hands. On the economic front, it has devastated the economies of the world, creating major uncertainties for countries and corporations, even preventing some of us from returning to our normal jobs and lives.

In this section we are focusing on how Covid-19 ignited substantial fires of anxiety and panic in those susceptible. Like all pandemics, it triggered uncertainty, from both a health and economic perspective. This particular pandemic created the greatest economic world-wide recession since the Great Depression, eclipsing, for example, the economic downturn of the previous decade.

It is unsurprising, therefore, that many of us have become so anxious. There would be something wrong if we were not, when facing down the twin barrels of a dangerous unpredictable virus and a creaking world economy. The pandemic tested our emotional resilience skills to the maximum. It was therefore inevitable that it would also increase the likelihood of all forms of anxiety, including panic attacks, phobias and general anxiety, especially the latter.

Such periods of enormous change particularly affect those who already crave and struggle for absolute control in their lives. This usually takes the form of seeking out absolute certainty, security, order or perfection. Since these demands are unachievable at the best of times, it was inevitable that for this group, levels of anxiety during the pandemic would increase. Some found themselves initially less anxious during the total lockdown as it contracted their world to a manageable size. When forced to leave the security of their homes and encounter a new, changed world, however, their anxiety levels rose. Many found themselves living in the watchtower, constantly hypervigilant and on edge, and scanning the environment for danger. This is what happened to Joe and there will be many readers who have lived through this pandemic who may find themselves empathizing with his story.

Joe's Story

Joe has been happily married to Mary for five years and is father to two school-age children. He is a middle-range manager with a large local company, while Mary works for a design company. All is going well in their lives, when the Covid-19 virus arrives into their world and Joe suddenly finds his life turned upside down. His company temporarily lays off all their staff, the schools close and Mary and himself find themselves socially locked down at home. Mary becomes the sole breadwinner but even she finds herself on reduced working hours and working from home. They are both suddenly under major economic and personal stress. Both struggle with trying to home-school their children, with Mary having the extra pressure of trying to complete her workload online.

Joe, who has always struggled with anxiety due to being a perfectionist, finds his fear and anxiety levels soaring. The sudden change throws him into a complete spin. He becomes increasingly anxious about everything. He worries about the virus attacking Mary or the kids or even himself, not to mention his mum and dad or siblings or in-laws. He becomes especially exercised, however, about his job, their financial security, even their very future as a unit.

Joe has always craved total certainty, perfection and security in all aspects of his life and prides himself on normally achieving these goals. Now all that certainty is gone and all he can see ahead is uncertainty. He begins to catastrophize wildly. Will he or any of his family get ill? Will someone close to him die? Will his company survive the crash? Will he have a job to go back to? Will they be able to pay their bills, especially their rent? What will the future hold for them all? All he can see ahead is darkness. He begins to see himself as a failure as he has not prepared sufficiently for such an eventuality and is now letting down his family.

The more anxious he becomes, the more physical symptoms he develops, with tension headaches, his stomach permanently in knots, struggling to sleep and difficulty concentrating on anything. He also struggles to pick up the phone or go online to seek out the relevant subsidies which the system has put in place to assist families like himself. Or to contact his bank or landlord to try to reschedule payments till the crisis abates. Instead, he finds himself gravitating towards sensational news feeds online, which support his view that the situation is only going to deteriorate further. His anxiety levels as a result continue to soar. He stops eating, loses weight and refuses to go out for daily exercise even though allowed to do so. Joe is clearly struggling to deal with this massive and sudden change in his life circumstances created by the Covid-19 pandemic.

While it is completely natural for anyone, including Joe, to be anxious during such periods, it is obvious that his anxiety levels are excessive. But why is this the case? The answer lies in his pre-existing beliefs and demands that he should be able to control all aspects of his life and that he is a failure if he is unable to achieve this impossible task. By seeking out 100 per cent certainty that neither he nor anyone close to him will become ill or die from the virus and that he must not lose his job, he is inevitably going to become increasingly anxious, as these demands are impossible to fulfil. Life is of course full of uncertainty, as we discussed in the previous chapter.

Joe is also catastrophizing completely, without any real proof that any of his fears are going to become reality. Yes, of course there is a possibility that any of the above could happen, but at present he has no proof that any one of them is in practice going to occur.

But let's see what happens when Joe decides to take out his pen and paper to silence his emotional mind and bring his rational mind and brain into the equation. He begins to apply the five-question pragmatic blueprint to his difficulties.

Here are Joe's answers:

1. **How is this situation making me feel?**

   'This sudden change in my circumstances is making me feel emotionally and physically extremely anxious.'

2. **What is it about this situation that is causing me to feel this way?**

   'I am feeling anxious as I am completely unsure or uncertain as to how this is going to work out. I have always craved certainty, to be in total control, but am now lost. Will I or some of my family get the virus and perhaps become extremely ill, or even die? Will I lose my job or income? I am also anxious as I am visualizing the very worst-case scenario all of the time, only seeking outside evidence to corroborate this. I can only see in my future illness, job loss, struggling to pay the rent and being thrown out of our home. Will my wife leave me in those circumstances? Will she see me, as I see myself, as a failure for not being able to protect my family?'

74

3. **What in my thinking is preventing me from dealing with this situation?**

    'I am demanding absolute certainty in a world where nothing is certain for any one of us. This makes no sense. I am also visualizing the worst-case scenario even though nothing has actually happened yet. I have simply been laid off, along with hundreds of thousands of others, as an emergency response to a public-health crisis. I am also demanding that neither I nor my family become ill with the virus, an equally impossible demand to deliver. Finally, I am being extremely self-critical of myself as not properly prepared for this emergency.'

4. **What in my behaviour is preventing me from dealing with this situation?**

    'My procrastination in relation to dealing with the situation is worsening the problems I am facing. I am especially creating difficulties for myself by not engaging with the bank and our landlord, and by not going online to claim any financial support available. Finally, I am wasting time instead, reading false and exaggerated social-media-driven news items, which are simply adding to my current woes.'

5. **How can I short-circuit my thinking and behavioural blocks to deal more effectively with this situation?**

    'In relation to my flawed thinking, I need to accept some harsh realities. Life at its core is both uncertain and insecure, as the whole world is finding out at present. There is also little point in spending my time and energy visualizing just how awful things might get. The reality is that with luck most or hopefully none of the outcomes that I am catastrophizing about will ever happen. Even if some of them do, I will cope with the help of my partner, wider family and friends. I have no other choice than to cope. I have a partner and two children to look after.

'I also need to let myself off the hook here. I am not a failure, nor indeed is anyone else for that matter. I am just a normal bloke, trying to deal with an extraordinary situation to the best of my abilities. It is natural that I am struggling. We are all struggling, both at an individual and community level. Some have described this pandemic as a war. Maybe it is time that I accepted that in war times are going to be difficult and challenging for everyone.

'In relation to my behaviour, it is time to take my head out of the sand and make the calls to banks and my landlord, who is actually a really good bloke, and also seek out online the support which I and my family are entitled to. After all, this is one of the benefits of being a citizen and paying my taxes!'

The good news is that by applying the above approaches, Joe finds it easier to deal with this extremely challenging period of change in his life. He does acquire a rental freeze from an understanding landlord, puts some loan repayments to the bank on hold and begins to claim the allowances his family are entitled to due to the crisis.

It still turns out to be an extremely difficult time for Joe and his family.

Both he and his family do become infected with the virus, but thankfully get over it within several weeks. His father is not so lucky and ends up on a ventilator in intensive care, but thankfully survives. When Joe does return to work, following some easing of restrictions, he and the rest of his work team find themselves initially on reduced hours. Mary, too, is on reduced hours, so finances continue to be tight.

There are many lessons to learn from his story. The first, and most obvious, is that there will be occasions in life, the Covid-19 pandemic being one of them, when there will be genuine reasons to be anxious. When there are real possibilities that negative outcomes may occur. When it is the situation that is abnormal and not us as individuals. The second is that for those who struggle with pre-existing anxiety, due to difficulties in coping with uncertainty, catastrophizing and self-rating, for example, scenarios such as Covid-19 can create chaos. The great news is that you, like Joe, can develop some pragmatic approaches which can greatly reduce your anxiety in such situations.

Joe is now looking at the Covid-19 pandemic and indeed many areas of his life in a new and increasingly pragmatic way. He is applying the above pragmatism exercise to many similar change scenarios occurring in his life. This has led to a great reduction in his anxiety and overall emotional distress. His company does survive and he thankfully returns to working full-time, sometimes from home and sometimes in the office, even if there are still some public-health restrictions being applied there.

Loneliness

Now let's meet Maeve, who is experiencing one of the commonest and least expressed fears of all human beings, namely the fear of loneliness. This can give rise to intense bouts of anxiety, such as the one she is facing now. In her case, as we shall see, loneliness is secondary to the sudden end of a long-term relationship. This can often be a key transitional moment of change in a person's life.

We tend to confuse the terms alone and lonely. You could, for example, be living alone and remain content and happy with life. Loneliness relates more to a pining for human relationships combined with a sense that you are somehow missing out on some key aspect of life. It is associated with a deep-seated inner longing to be loved, and a belief that you are a failure if this is not happening. It can be extremely damaging to your physical and mental health.

The commonest fear of loneliness relates to the world of personal relationships. Men and women are not designed to live their lives alone. Although some do so and thrive, they are the exception. For the rest of us, the threat of loneliness might be our greatest fear. Fears about being left alone and lonely can occur at any stage in our lives. There are key transitional periods, however, such as a relationship break-up or the death of a partner or loved one, that can especially trigger this emotion.

Such periods of change tend to trigger uncertainty, catastrophizing and often profound self-rating, all three of which commonly underlie anxiety.

There are countless people who will empathize and see themselves in this story. You may have lost your long-term friend or life partner and are simply bereft and don't know where to turn. You may have just experienced a relationship break-up with someone special. You may have been unlucky and have so far struggled to meet that special person and feel anxious that you never will. I hope that, whatever the underlying reason is, you will find hope and inspiration in Maeve's story and how she uses our pragmatic blueprint to reshape her life.

Maeve's Story

Maeve is a thirty-seven-year-old primary school teacher, who has been living with her partner Jerry for the previous nine years. They met at a party when she was in her late twenties and there was an instant attraction. Jerry works as a business executive in a busy multinational company. Within six months they were living together and, in her mind, this was the man she would be spending the rest of her life with. For the first five or six years, their relationship went smoothly, although Maeve found his frequent absences for business trips abroad upsetting. They live in an apartment in the city and avail themselves of the latter's many amenities. Maeve herself comes from the country but has quickly learned to enjoy what the city has to offer. She loves her job as a teacher and her life in general is very fulfilling.

As Maeve approaches her thirty-fifth birthday, however, she begins to notice how many of her friends are making long-term commitments or plans to start a family. As a close friend comments, time is moving on and if Maeve wants to have a family, it is time to start making some moves. She begins to gently broker the subject with Jerry, but to her surprise and disappointment hits unexpected resistance. Jerry is completely against either making their current set-up more official or starting a family. Are they not happy and content with their lives as they are? What is marriage, for example, but a piece of paper? Has he not seen many of his friends arrive in the divorce courts? As for children, it would be impossible to fit them into their busy lives. The more Maeve tries to change his mind, the more withdrawn he becomes. Eventually, she decides to leave things as they are and ceases discussing the matter. She really loves this man and if this is the price she will have to pay, she is prepared to accept it.

Two years later, however, a bombshell arrives. Jerry returns from a seemingly normal business meeting abroad to announce that he has met someone at one of his meetings. He has decided to leave Maeve and move abroad to live with his new partner. She tries to remonstrate with him. Is he sure that this is not simply a fling, a brief attraction? How could he just throw away nine years of their relationship, seemingly at the drop of a hat? But Jerry is adamant, and then reveals that he has been seeing this person for over a year. He also believes that their own relationship has been going steadily downhill for over a year. It is clear to him that they both want different things out of life. It is best to separate and go their own ways. Within a month, he moves abroad and Maeve is on her own.

Devastated by this sudden change in her life, she experiences a rollercoaster of emotions, from initial hurt, anger and sadness to overwhelming feelings of anxiety and panic. With the assistance of some friends, she begins to deal with the sadness and even rationalizes her initial anger and hurt. But nothing prepares her for the waves of anxiety, which threaten to overwhelm her. Or the overwhelming feelings of loneliness which emerge following his departure and the worry that she will be left like this. Her anxiety levels soar and within eight weeks she is physically and emotionally exhausted.

Her lovely ordered world is now in tatters. She is uncertain about future personal relationships. She begins to visualize the worst. She is now thirty-seven and increasingly unlikely to meet anyone, especially someone like Jerry, who, despite everything, she still loves. The more she examines herself in the mirror, the more she sees the early signs of ageing. Nobody will be interested in her at this stage, especially when they realize that she has come from a failed long-term relationship. It is hopeless. She now can't even look forward to having children either, so may end up completely alone. All she sees stretching ahead are years of loneliness and possibly bitterness over all she has lost.

Maeve also constantly berates herself for her current state of loneliness. Has she not created her current problems by putting too much pressure on Jerry? If she does end up alone and lonely for the rest of her life, does it suggest that she is a failure and of little value to herself or others? All she sees on her social-media outlets are videos of close friends in wonderful relationships looking forward to meaningful lives with their partners. Is she going to be the ugly duckling if left on her own alone?

She retreats into herself, relying more on bottles of wine to assuage her gnawing anxiety. She struggles at work, but manages to hide her difficulties from colleagues, family members and friends. She shrugs off the break-up as 'one of those things' and, notably, never shares her feelings of loneliness. She eats junk food, puts on a significant amount of weight, dumps her exercise regimens and finds her sleep patterns disrupted.

Deep down, she knows she ought to be visiting a counsellor to deal with the separation, but she keeps putting this off. What difference will it make? She avoids any potential subsequent relationship hook-ups, set up by well-meaning friends, and refuses to enter the online dating scene. In her mind, it is over. She had her chance and blew it! She is also terrified of any future commitments, having been so badly burned on this occasion. The loneliness, however, increasingly gnaws away at her insides. Her anxiety levels increase further. She finds herself trapped between the fear of any future commitment and the looming spectre of lifelong loneliness.

What is happening to Maeve is that she is becoming emotionally and physically anxious, unable to deal with the uncertainty this break-up has created in her life. She is seeking complete reassurance that she will not end up alone and lonely. Maeve is also spending most of her time catastrophizing about how awful life without someone special is going to be and negatively self-rating herself for allowing this state of loneliness to arise. Her behaviours are also not helping. By eating poorly, putting on weight, ceasing exercise and not sharing her emotional distress with others or a counsellor, she is adding to her difficulties. Her decision to block out further romantic possibilities prevent her from feeling any further pain. But they also remove the possibility of future long-term relationships, which might in turn reduce her risks of long-term loneliness. She is becoming a self-fulfilling prophecy.

Let's see what happens when Maeve, on the advice of a friend, decides to analyse her current situation on paper, using the five-question pragmatic blueprint detailed earlier.

Here is Maeve's blueprint:

1. **How is this situation making me feel?**
   'Jerry's departure from our relationship and the ensuing loneliness is making me feel emotionally and physically anxious.'

2. **What is it about this situation that is making me feel this way?**

'I am feeling anxious, unsure and uncertain as to how all of this is going to end. Will I ever meet anyone like Jerry again? I can only see a bleak future in front of me. I am in my late thirties, with the physical bloom of youth fading, so am unlikely to meet someone whom I could love again. I only see a future shorn of a partner or children, a bleak place where I will end up lonely and alone. I know that if this happens, I will see myself as a failure, useless and of little value to myself or others.'

3. **What in my thinking is preventing me from dealing with this situation?**

    'I am demanding absolute certainty that I do not finish up alone and lonely, with no partner or children. I am catastrophizing as to how awful my future is going to be if this does happen. I am also constantly judging myself as a failure for allowing this to occur.'

4. **What in my behaviour is preventing me from dealing with this situation?**

    'I am trying to hide the way I feel from family and close friends, refusing to share my distress with them. I am also avoiding attending a counsellor. My current lifestyle is clearly not helping. My weight gain from junk food and my alcohol binges are just worsening the way I feel. I am also avoiding the world of dating, for fear of being unsuccessful or getting hurt and having to re-experience this pain and distress.'

5. **How can I short-circuit my thinking and behavioural blocks to deal more effectively with this issue?**

    'In relation to my thinking, I need to accept that nothing in life is absolutely certain and that none of us is ever sure of what life has in store for us. Yes, there is a risk or chance that I may end up alone and lonely, but is that risk not there for everyone? There can never be complete certainty, for example, when any of us enter a relationship, as to whether it will work out or finish in tears. If all of us demanded otherwise, nobody would ever enter a relationship. Re-entering the dating scene will obviously involve the same risks and uncertainties, but I cannot run away from such risks as they are the realities of life. I either take the chance, or finish up alone and lonely, and I know where that leads!

'It might be more useful to challenge my catastrophizing as to how awful a life of loneliness might be, and use my time more constructively instead, by coming up with solutions to my current dilemma.

'I am also being extremely hard and cruel in terms of how I describe myself as a person. I am not a failure or worthless or useless simply because I am experiencing a period of loneliness. Rather, I am a unique, special person, whom I must learn to accept unconditionally. If I want to rate something about myself, perhaps it should be my behaviour, where I am putting my head in the sand and not actively dealing with the situation.

'In relation to my behaviour, I am clearly going to have a serious chat with myself about my diet, lack of exercise and over-reliance on wine. All of these are just making me feel even worse about myself. Things around here are going to have to change!

'I have to be more honest with family and friends, share my worries and concerns about loneliness and seek support and encouragement from them. I may even have to consider counselling. But most of all, I have to engage again in the dating scene, even though the thought fills me with fear and anxiety. I am still a young woman in the prime of her life and with much to give. But it is up to me to put myself out there, in the hope of meeting someone new to share my life and dreams with. It will not be easy, and there will be many setbacks, but the prize is worth fighting for.'

Let's now discover what actually happens when Maeve – following this pragmatic analysis of her current difficulties with loneliness – puts the above into action.

She rolls up her sleeves and executes some major lifestyle changes. Out go the wine and junk food and in comes a strict dietary and exercise regimen. Within three months she has lost weight, is glowing with health and feels better physically and emotionally. She shares with family members and close friends just how lonely and distressed she has become. She is overwhelmed by their love and support and no longer feels she requires counselling. Some share privately with her how they too have experienced periods of loneliness, usually for a similar reason, and how distressing they found them to be.

Maeve, with the assistance of her close friend, begins to date again. To her surprise, she enjoys many of the interactions which occur, even if quite a few of them come to nothing. She is now increasingly acceptant that relationships fail, not people, and that sometimes things work out really well and sometimes not. That's life. It is up to her to reduce the chances of finishing up alone and lonely, by engaging with this world. She also accepts that there is little point in being hard on herself if this does happen, as she is doing her best to ensure it does not occur. Even if this were to happen, it will not change who she is, a unique, special person who has learned to accept herself unconditionally.

Maeve has not yet met that special somebody, but she is no longer struggling with her fear of loneliness. And there is someone . . . interesting!

PART THREE

FRUSTRATION

5. Why Change Can Make You Frustrated

Do you respond to some significant period of change by becoming emotionally frustrated? Instead of becoming fearful, worried or anxious, do you become easily frustrated, even irritable, with the arrival of a new situation in your life over which you may have little or no control? If so, you may wonder why.

Suppose your emotional response to not getting a job interview, which in the previous section might have been anxiety, is instead one of frustration or annoyance. 'Can't they see how much I have to offer?' 'Why did they ask me those stupid questions at the interview?' 'What did those questions have to do with the job I was being interviewed for?' 'It's just nonsense – clearly they have a poor interviewing panel. I know I did a good interview, and in my mind was obviously the best person for the post.' 'Why can't they see matters the way I see them?'

The difficulty with the emotion of frustration is that it can often prevent you from dealing with the problematic change which has presented itself. The reality of life is that change is going to regularly rear its head and present you with ongoing periods of disruption. If you continue to react with this emotion, you will find such periods of change extremely challenging indeed.

The good news is that you can, as with anxiety, develop a pragmatic blueprint to better manage such periods, and we will be exploring this in the next chapter. Let's first explore why some common pitfalls in relation to your thinking and behaviour may explain why you are struggling so much with this emotion.

The Importance of Discomfort

Life is tough, a constant battle for survival, as many of us can attest. There will always be those wonderfully joyous occasions when everything seems to be running smoothly. Alas, there will also be significant periods of hassle, disturbance and discomfort. All of us, on occasion, become frustrated during such periods, wishing them to be different. Discomfort is, and always will be, an integral part of human existence, with the majority of us building into our lives coping mechanisms to deal with it. Discomfort is a fact of life, which most of us accept and simply get on with. However, some of us can really struggle with this harsh reality, and waste a lot of time and energy trying to avoid it. This can in turn lead to periods of intense frustration as we demand that this should not be the case. Why are we being asked to accept and deal with this discomfort? Why are others not experiencing it, whilst we are?

Periods of change are especially challenging for those who struggle with discomfort. For change usually means that your normal routines have been disrupted or disturbed. You are no longer in control, as events may have overtaken you. The Covid-19 pandemic is a good example of how life can suddenly turn normal routines upside down. All of us struggled with the sudden complete disruption to our lives, the social isolation, the absence of friends, the inability to enjoy normal socialization, sport and so many other activities which enrich our lives. While others may have become extremely anxious, you may have noticed that you became intensely frustrated instead. You may have found yourself railing against the situation, especially in the beginning, perhaps becoming irritable and moody in the process. Why am I having to put up with the discomfort of having to stay in all the time? Why can't I visit my friends or slip over to a neighbour's house for a small party? The reality being, of course, that the pandemic was challenging you to accept the discomfort of such restrictions for the higher goal of keeping vulnerable citizens alive.

Periods of change can lead to significant discomfort. Failure to manage such periods can therefore lead to emotions of intense frustration. If you can relate to this, it is likely that you, too, may be trying to dodge the discomfort that often follows in the wake of such times of change. But why do you respond this way? The answer lies in your irrational belief systems, discussed previously. You have, over time, developed an irrational belief or demand that you should not have to suffer discomfort. And that is often where the trouble for you begins!

The pragmatic approach to discomfort is that disturbance, hassle or being knocked out of your comfort zone is a part of life and a reality which you cannot dodge, no matter how much you wish this not to be the case. I often use the two words 'Hello, life' to good-humouredly describe this reality. Life since the beginning of time has been tough, uncompromising and full of discomfort. It is unlikely to change any time soon, so it's better to accept this reality and move on!

The Role of Instant Gratification

Another important reason why you may respond to change with frustration is that you may struggle with the concept of delayed gratification. This can be simply put as 'I want it now'! Suppose you are given a box of chocolates. You have two choices. The first is to have a few and then put the box away to enjoy them at a later date, perhaps with family members or friends. The second choice is to guzzle them all immediately, while enjoying a movie. Which would you do?

If you battle with frustration, chances are that you will most likely take the second option. To put them away would mean denying yourself the immediate pleasure buzz that such a chocolate orgy would produce. I might suggest to you that delaying this pleasure in part for the purpose of enjoying it in the future would be preferable and better for your waistline. Your answer might be 'I don't want to put off enjoying them till later, I want them now!'

This concept links in with the previous section on discomfort. If you delay, then you will suffer the discomfort of being unable to scoff the box. Your natural tendency therefore may veer towards instant gratification.

The pragmatic approach to your demand for instant gratification will involve an acceptance that constantly trying to achieve this demand will cause you to struggle for two reasons. The first is that life may often remove this as an option, whether you like it or not. The second is that you will find it much harder to cope with periods of significant change if you are unable to accept the concept of 'short-term pain for long-term gain'. This is where you teach yourself the skill of looking at the broader picture, being prepared, if necessary, to deny yourself something in the here and now in order to achieve a more substantial goal in the future. Applying this concept to the recent pandemic really brings this home. The long-term goal was to protect the vulnerable in our society, safeguard our own health and that of our loved ones and to safeguard future employment possibilities. The short-term pain was to accept the social isolation and lockdown measures. Thankfully the vast majority of us accepted this reality and behaved accordingly.

Life will present you with multiple opportunities to put this pragmatic insight into practice, as we will explore later.

The Situation Must Change

Another common reason for becoming frustrated is the irrational belief that it is up to situations and indeed life itself to change, rather than you! This can lead to the irrational demand that 'the situation must change, not me'. This once again feeds back into the demand that you should not have to put up with discomfort, discussed already.

We all find ourselves struggling with sudden periods of change, where something happens, often unexpectedly, which challenges our capacity to cope. You might be someone who is transferred at short notice, into a different section of a company, and find yourself at loggerheads immediately with a new manager, unhappy with the change. You might be a teacher having to take over a second class when a colleague becomes suddenly ill. Or someone who has been turned down for a promotion or pay rise at work. You might be a student who is finding a new subject at college more difficult than anticipated. The list of possibilities is endless. All will lead to disturbance and hassle.

Suppose your emotional response is to become frustrated, however, because you believe that it is up to others to do something about your new situation. That it is not your responsibility to sort the issue out, but rather someone else's. Or that the situation should simply not be presenting itself at all. That life should not be giving you this unexpected disturbance, hassle or discomfort. You may find your behavioural responses to this demand to be equally inappropriate. Some of you may already see yourself in these beliefs and demands. That it is up to other people to change, not you. How many of you can easily relate to the intense frustration which arises when such demands are not being met by people, situations and indeed on occasion by life itself?

As with discomfort, many of us can easily pick up such irrational beliefs and demands as we pass through life. It is not so easy to recognize and accept them, unless we are truly honest with ourselves. The good news is that you can develop new approaches and skills which will allow you to better challenge, and manage, such situations of change.

The pragmatic approach is that people, situations and indeed life itself have absolutely no intention of changing to suit you, even if such a possibility seems extremely attractive. You will be waiting a while, for example, for the Inland Revenue to send you a rebate cheque in the post just because you believe that you are paying too much tax! If we take some of the above cases, the new boss is not going to suddenly change personality to accommodate you. Nor are you going to change your boss's mind as to that promotion or bonus simply because you believe you deserve it. Nor as a student are you going to be told to skip the difficult parts of the course, just because you are finding them tough. You get the message! It would be wonderful of course if all of the above did happen in practice, but if you are waiting, it may be a long wait.

Another important pragmatic reality, following on from above, is that sometimes in life you will encounter situations where even if you are open and prepared to make changes, it will not be possible to change the outcome. In such situations you have to accept and adapt to this reality or else remain incredibly frustrated.

The pragmatic message is pretty clear here. If situations are to improve for the better, the chances are that it will be up to you and you alone to bring about the relevant changes. This will mean deciding to change what you can, and on other occasions accepting what you can't!

The Role of Your Behaviour

It is important to note that how you respond behaviourally when change makes you frustrated can often add to the problem. There are two common behaviour responses which can be problematic.

Destructive Behaviour

If you are someone who struggles with frustration, it is likely that you may see yourself in some of the following behaviours. The most common of these which you may recognize, is irritability. This is where you find yourself being bad-tempered or short with others, including loved ones, friends or colleagues. You may notice that you are constantly speaking angrily about being asked to manage a situation which is guaranteed to bring you hassle or discomfort.

Sometimes this irritability can lead to more destructive behaviours, such as being aggressive on the road, even road rage or picking verbal fights with others. Or being boorish in restaurants.

Or caustic on social-media sites. Or drinking more to cope with your frustration levels.

The pragmatic approach to such behaviours is that they are not achieving their objective. You are still going to have to manage the new situation in which you find yourself. This is not going to change, despite your behaviour. Nor is it going to prevent you experiencing discomfort. All that it is doing is harming yourself. Human beings do not respond well to others being constantly irritable, short or moody with them. They tend to react negatively. Nor does such negative behaviour in restaurants, queues or on the road in any way improve your current dilemma. And neither does excessive alcohol consumption.

Procrastinating Behaviour

A second common behavioural response to frustration is procrastination, discussed in the previous chapter, where you put off dealing with a situation. This is because you are unable to convince yourself to accept the discomfort involved and make changes to deal with the new situation. You might be frustrated, for example, that you are a young person attending college who wants to get out there and enjoy the good life but instead are struggling to prepare for an upcoming exam. You know that eventually you are going to have to sit this exam. However, there are so many other 'temptations' that draw you away from doing the hard work deemed necessary. You keep putting off studying till the last minute, and then find yourself desperately cramming to catch up, with the possibility of having to repeat the exams rapidly looming in your rear-view mirror.

The pragmatic approach to such behaviour is to ask yourself whether a delay in coming to terms with the cause and consequences of the change in question is only adding to your woes.

It is the classic case of short-term pain versus long-term gain discussed above. You can either experience the discomfort now or later. The choice is yours!

6. How to Manage Your 'Change' Frustration

In the previous chapter, we examined why change can make you frustrated and how your behaviours add to this. Now let's see if pragmatism could assist you to overcome these obstacles and reduce your change-driven frustration.

The Pragmatic Approach to Frustration

A pragmatic approach to change-driven frustration will involve, as previously discussed, learning how to deal with discomfort, accepting short-term pain for long-term gain and realizing that situations tend not to change just because we wish them to. It is *you* that will often need to change. It will also challenge whether the destructive or procrastinating behaviours already detailed are assisting us or preventing you from dealing with the underlying causes of your frustration. Let's apply our five-question pragmatic blueprint, detailed in chapter two, to assist Andrew, who struggles with frustration and who in his own words describes himself as a 'talented procrastinator'.

The Tasks We Want to Avoid

All of us can relate in some ways to Andrew. There are some specific tasks or assignments that we 'dread' and keep putting off. It may be cutting the grass, doing the ironing or sorting out our financial affairs, for example. Our natural tendency is to avoid or put off such jobs or assignments. The reality, of course, is that these tasks do not simply go away, but will keep staring us in the face till we reluctantly face the music and deal with them.

For some of us, including Andrew, this tendency to procrastinate is associated with intense emotions of frustration almost becoming a way of life. For this group, any sudden change in their day-to-day circumstances which will involve an extra or unexpected amount of work will trigger this emotion and cause significant irritation. You may see yourself in his story!

Andrew's Story

Andrew, a vice-principal of his school, is asked unexpectedly by the principal to complete an important assignment within the following month. He has always suffered from frustration, as his long-suffering partner Marian and his two teenage children could attest. Even as a teenager, he was renowned for having a short fuse. In college he ducked and weaved his way through his assignments and exams, with a lot of last-minute cramming to get through. He carries this emotion into his job. As a vice-principal he is popular with his fellow teachers but again is renowned for having a short fuse if things are not going his way. It was inevitable, therefore, that this request would trigger his go-to emotion of frustration and that he would revert to his usual behaviour of procrastination, delaying the task and expressing his anger to anyone who would listen!

Let's see what happens when Andrew decides instead to apply our pragmatic blueprint to his current situation.

This was Andrew's blueprint:

1. **How is this situation making me feel?**
'My emotion is frustration.'

2. **What is it about this situation that is causing me to feel this way?**
'Why should I have to put up with the hassle and disturbance of this task, which I find boring in the extreme? Why did he delegate this assignment at the last moment to me of all people? I could be doing so many other tasks which I would find more interesting and rewarding. Why does my principal not see things the way I see them and pass the job on to another colleague?'

3. **What in my thinking is preventing me from dealing with this situation?**
'It is probably to do with my demand that I should not have to put up with the discomfort and hassle of this task. And that my principal should see matters the same way and pass the task on to someone else.'

4. **What in my behaviour is preventing me from dealing with this situation?**
'I am doing my usual "Andrew trick" and delaying and procrastinating the task till time runs out. I usually find myself frantically trying to finish it at the last minute. I am also, as usual, irritable with those around me as I am so frustrated with being given this task in the first place.'

5. **How could I short-circuit my thinking and behavioural blocks to deal more effectively with this situation?**
   'I have to get realistic here. The task will have to be finished, one way or the other, so I must accept that this will involve hard work and discomfort. The chances of my principal changing his mind and giving it to someone else are slim to nil. I will have to therefore deal with my own discomfort and simply get on with it, if I wish to keep him happy and off my back.

   'In relation to my behaviour, I need to stop being irritable and moaning constantly to everyone around me. I need to stop procrastinating and perhaps instead break the task into smaller chunks and gradually tick off each chunk. This will mean that I will get the job completed with a lot less stress in the time available, instead of my usual last-minute rush. This might leave me more time on the football pitch training the lads, which is really more my thing.'

This pragmatic analysis allows Andrew to understand why he has become frustrated with the situation in the first place, how his behaviour has worsened matters and, most importantly, how to change his thinking and behaviour to manage it better.

As a result, he decides to attack his assignment. He begins by setting a personal deadline of three weeks, dividing the task into thirds. He completes a third each week with ease, and still has time to enjoy other areas of his life. He is able to complete and hand in his assignment ahead of time, with minimal stress.

Now let's meet Stephen, Zoe and Paul, all struggling with frustration as a response to some problematic change in their lives. You may see yourself in some of their stories.

The Parent v. Young Adult Phase

Let's begin with Stephen, who is struggling to come to terms with a decision made by his daughter Maria with which he fundamentally disagrees. This is a common scenario, familiar to us all, namely disagreements between parents and young adult children.

How many of you can relate to this scenario, whether as a parent or a young adult? You may be going through just such a situation at present. There can be frustration on both sides, depending on how the parties involved view the situation. This is inevitable. Parents often forget that their job as a parent ceases at eighteen, following which they become mentors or advisors. Because of this, they often seek to overrule decisions made by their young adult children. The latter equally forget that their parents are only doing what they think is best for their adult children. This can lead to significant emotional distress for one or the other.

The period between eighteen to thirty is often one of great change, especially for the young adult, as they struggle to come to terms and cope with the adult world in which they are now residing. Young people slowly but surely become increasingly mature and adult as they advance through their twenties. It can often, therefore, take some time for them to decide what they really want to do with the rest of their lives. Sometimes this can happen in the early to mid-twenties, and sometimes later. This understanding is important, as around these periods young adults may decide to take some significant changes in direction. Some parents, like Stephen, with the best of intentions, can struggle emotionally with these sudden periods of change. For those who struggle with frustration, such periods can especially challenge their view of the world. Let's see how pragmatism assists Stephen in coming to terms with his emotional responses to his daughter's sudden decision to change her career in her mid-twenties.

Stephen's Story

Stephen, who is in his early fifties, is in a long-term relationship with Elaine. They have three children, of whom the eldest, Maria, is twenty-four. Relationships between Maria, her two brothers and their parents have always been good, even if she finds her dad to be inflexible in many areas. She loves him dearly, but on occasion finds him 'trying'!

Maria, who has a sunny disposition, has always been unsure as to what she wants to do with her life. She drifts into doing an arts degree, with the vague notion of doing primary-school teaching. Her dad, Stephen, is delighted with this decision as he is a school principal himself. Her mother Elaine is shrewder, suggesting on one occasion that Maria should take her time, on completion of her degree, to reassess what she wants to do long term with her life.

Maria hates the college course she is doing, quickly realizing that she is like a square peg in a round hole. She has always been a creative, more hands-on person, and finds the subjects chosen are strangling this side of her nature. She hates letting her dad down, and so following a chat with her mum decides to finish the course.

By the time she has done so, she is twenty-four and in a serious relationship with Simon, who is an artist. He suggests a change to doing something more creative. With his assistance, she subsequently discovers wood-turning and an innate talent for creating beautiful designs out of bog wood.

She decides to postpone any decision to become a teacher and to focus instead on furthering her new-found talent.

She is unprepared for the onslaught from her dad, who is bitterly disappointed that she has not progressed into a postgraduate teaching course as per her original idea. Matters are not helped by the relationship between her partner Simon and Stephen, which is strained, to say the least. Stephen sees Simon as the reason that his daughter had made this sudden change of plan.

Elaine does her best to smooth out the relationship between her husband and Maria but to no avail. Her husband is simply not for turning, so Maria moves in with Simon, shutting down links with her dad, hurt by his reactions to both her partner and her new career.

As for Stephen, frustration levels mount as he rails against Maria's decision. How could she throw away all that education to mess around instead with pieces of wood? Why would she not progress to have a good career and a quality of life as a teacher, which in his mind would be much more rewarding? Can she not see that her dad has more life experience and that she should be listening to him? As for Simon, the less said the better. Even his name triggers intense frustration and irritability as he is the one facilitating this sudden change in his daughter's life, which Stephen considers so negative.

Stephen's frustration, an emotion which those close to him were used to experiencing, spills over into other areas of his life. At work, he finds himself becoming more irritable with colleagues, students and parents. It takes less and less to set him off on a rant. At home, he becomes increasingly irritable with Elaine and their other two teenage children.

He refuses to keep in contact with Maria, even though he misses her greatly. Eventually it is Elaine who pulls him up sharply on this, by asking him one simple question: 'Are you more interested in the happiness of your daughter, or having your own way in relation to her life decisions?' This insightful comment shocks him into reassessing the situation.

Now let's see what happens when Stephen, with Elaine's assistance, decides to apply the five-question pragmatic blueprint to his current situation. He finds that this approach allows his more rational, problem-solving side to come to the surface.

Here is Stephen's blueprint:

1. **How is this situation making me feel?**
   'This decision by Maria to take a different direction in her life is triggering intense frustration.'

2. **What is it about this situation that is causing me to feel this way?**
   'I am feeling frustrated, as I've been asked to accept a completely new situation in both her and my lives. She is choosing to ignore the effort and money it took to finish her degree, and not using it wisely to enter a career which has given me such fulfilment. Why is she not listening to me, her father, with so much life experience behind me, choosing instead to listen to the advice of Simon, who seems to be doing nothing important with his life?

   'Her decision not to follow the road that I have suggested is making me experience discomfort, as I like things to be the way that I feel they should be!'

3. **What in my thinking is preventing me from dealing with this situation?**

'I am demanding (probably irrationally) that I should not have to put up with the discomfort of others, in this case Maria, not listening to my advice. I am demanding that she must see things as I do and continue with her education to become a teacher, rather than wasting time on bog-wood carving! I am also demanding that she finds a different partner, as I believe that Simon is not good for her. Once again, she should be listening to my advice on this issue.'

4. **What in my behaviour is preventing me from dealing with this situation?**

'In terms of my behaviour, I am being irritable and bad-tempered with everyone, my work colleagues and Elaine and the two boys. I am purposely avoiding making contact with Maria, instead of trying to keep the relationship going and resolve matters between us.'

5. **How can I short-circuit my thinking and behavioural blocks to deal more effectively with this situation?**

'In relation to my flawed thinking, I need to rethink some of my demands, which, on reflection, do seem completely unreasonable. I am refusing to accept that Maria is now a mature young adult, entitled to make whatever changes she wishes in her own life and that I have no right to insist that she does otherwise. I am entitled as her dad to express my concerns about any course of action which she might take, but not to impose my view of the world on her.

'I need to listen more to Elaine, who argues that Maria has always had a creative streak in her, which is finally coming to the fore. I have no right to decide who Maria meets or falls in love with. Come to think of it, I am not sure Elaine's dad was over-excited when I swept her off her feet! Maria has the right to choose who she wants to spend the rest of her life with, and frankly it is no business of mine to interfere.

'It is clear that I have several options open to me. If I continue to travel down my current road, then I may lose my daughter and even potential grandchildren over time. I would also be denying Elaine this relationship, which is so important to her. Is this not a selfish decision on my behalf? The more sensible option is to re-connect with Maria and establish some common ground, allowing all of us to move forward with our lives.

'In relation to my unhelpful behaviour, there is clearly a need for me challenge it. Is my bad-tempered behaviour and irritability with Elaine and the two boys, not to mention those with whom I interact with at work, actually sorting out the situation, or making matters worse? Clearly the latter. It is my decision to avoiding meeting up with Maria and refusing to accept Simon into our lives that is causing much of the current difficulties. I am the one who is going to have to make some changes if I wish to resolve this crisis.'

Let's discover what happens when Stephen decides, following this pragmatic analysis of his daughter's sudden change of direction, to put this blueprint into action.

He begins with a frank conversation with Elaine, and together they work out a strategy to manage the situation. Elaine has an initial conversation with Maria and acts as a go-between. Maria then meets up with Stephen, who apologizes for his behaviour to date. He admits that he has been completely wrong in insisting that she enters the teaching world if she believes that her real strength lies in her creativity. They have an emotional conversation, as she explains that all she wants from her dad is his love and support. It ends in a warm embrace and the beginning of a new adult relationship between them.

Maria also reveals how her new partner, Simon, has been at the forefront of encouraging her to rekindle her relationship with her dad, whom he greatly respects. Stephen admits that he has not given Simon a chance so far as he has been blaming him for Maria's change of direction. He vows to do everything in his power to create a new bond with him. If this is the man his daughter has chosen as her partner, then the least he can do is welcome him in as part of their family. Over time, both men get closer and discover mutual areas of interest, both following the same football team.

Maria's work is now increasingly in demand, with Stephen truly appreciating her creative gift. Simon and Maria rapidly become an important part of their family unit, with Stephen now accepting that they must be allowed to live their lives as they see fit.

But the real game-changer for Stephen is his decision to pragmatically challenge his demand that everyone else must change, not him, and his tendency to be irritable and bad-tempered with others. He finds this task challenging, but over months discovers his frustration levels rapidly diminishing and, as a result, his life running more smoothly. He is now ready for whatever new life changes come his way. And they do, in the form of a new grandson, two years later, who rapidly becomes the apple of his eye. It really was a case of short-term pain for long-term gain.

Workplace Restructuring

Now let's catch up with Zoe, who is experiencing another common scenario, familiar to many of us, namely a period of major workplace restructuring. Significant numbers of us spend much of our days and weeks at work. We become accustomed to, and comfortable with, set routines and patterns. The workplace, however, like life, can be fickle and prone to periods of change and upheaval. As we have already explored, it is not these periods of change which create difficulties for us, but rather how we interpret them, as is the case for Zoe, who reacts by becoming extremely frustrated. There will be many reading this who will empathize with her story.

> *Zoe's Story*
>
> Zoe, in her early thirties, works in a large, vibrant multinational company. She is regarded by her peers as a fast-track, upwardly moving executive, clearly being groomed for greater things. She also has a reputation as someone with low frustration tolerance levels, becoming quickly irritable and short-fused if those around her don't reach her standards of perfection. She is in a long-term relationship with Sean, who has a quiet, laid-back personality. Even he on occasion finds himself on the receiving end of her ire when work is not progressing well. Overall, however, Zoe is happy with her life, both at home and at work.
>
> But then her world suddenly implodes as, due to financial constraints, her head office in the States closes down and they restructure different parts of their global operation, with Zoe's workplace not being spared. Massive changes are introduced overnight. She finds herself in a completely restructured section, with a retinue of new staff, and presented

with totally different sets of objectives. She rapidly finds herself out of her normal comfort zone.

Her new team firstly requires retraining, which causes her intense frustration. Why is she having to spend her time babysitting this group, whilst trying to bring them up to speed? Shouldn't she be free to do what she prefers most, which is to forward-plan future projects?

But worse is to come. Head office then parachutes in 'one of their own' to run the section. Zoe and her new boss are immediately at loggerheads over the direction their section should be taking. He is conservative by nature, whereas Zoe is a calculated risk-taker. Her frustration levels rise. She becomes short-tempered and irritable with both her boss and her colleagues. Nor does Sean escape her wrath. Zoe begins to imbibe more wine each evening, which unleashes her aggressive side. Their relationship becomes rockier as Sean struggles to live with her behaviour. She simultaneously picks up a speeding fine for blasting down the motorway in an attempt to release her frustration levels.

At work, matters deteriorate further. Her boss, fed up with her constant challenging of his decisions, assigns her a project which he knows she will find dull and demands a short delivery deadline. Zoe groans when she sees the assignment, realizing immediately that she will find it extremely boring. As is her normal behaviour in such cases, she procrastinates, purposely delaying the assignment, choosing instead to seek out more interesting challenges. This sets her on a collision course with her new boss.

Zoe's life has suddenly changed for the worse, with her normal organized world in danger of falling apart. Her mounting frustration and accompanying behaviour are also putting at risk her current role in the organization and more importantly her relationship with Sean.

Let's examine what happens when Zoe, on the advice of a close friend, decides to apply pragmatism to her situation, courtesy of our five-question blueprint.

Here is Zoe's blueprint:

1. **How is this situation making me feel?**
   'This change in my workplace is making me feel intensely frustrated.'

2. **What is it about this situation that is causing me to feel this way?**
   'I am frustrated at being asked to accept a completely new situation at work. I have had to change departments, train new staff, accept a boss whom I believe is too conservative and take on boring assignments. Why should I be asked to put up with all this change, hassle and disturbance to my previously organized working life? Why me? Surely others are better suited to this section? Why can't head office see that this is not a sensible use of my talents and experience?'

3. **What in my thinking is preventing me from dealing with this situation?**
   'I am demanding (probably irrationally) that I should not have to suffer any disturbance or discomfort. I am also demanding that decisions made at global and head-office level should be put to one side because these decisions do not suit me. And further, that my colleagues and new boss should change personality to suit me. This is clearly daft when I see it written down in

my own words! Above all, I am refusing to accept that changes made at global level will have consequences for everyone and that I am no different.'

4. **What in my behaviour is preventing me from dealing with this situation?**

    'In terms of my behaviour, I am being irritable and bad-tempered with everyone at work and with poor Sean, who has experienced a lot of my irritability and sup-pressed annoyance at home. I am drinking too much, which is making matters worse. I am delaying beginning my latest project, as it is boring, but this is only putting further pressure on myself over the next few weeks. And as for the speeding fine, that speaks for itself.'

5. **How can I short-circuit my thinking and behavioural blocks to deal more effectively with this situation?**

    'In relation to my flawed thinking, I need to accept some harsh realities. Global companies are not going to alter their policies simply because I am not happy with such changes. Nor are my boss or colleagues going to change any time soon. And why should they? I couldn't see myself changing if the shoe was on the other foot. I also have to accept that disturbance and discomfort are a part of life and I, like everyone else, cannot dodge them. Am I really justified in insisting that this boring task which I keep putting off should be done by someone else?

    'The only person who can clearly change in relation to all of these matters is myself. I have three clear choices here. I could accept the current situation and put up with it, hoping to be eventually moved to a new section. I could make some unofficial approaches to personnel or personal contacts in head office to see if such a change could be facilitated. Or I could seek out new pastures further afield.

'In relation to my unhelpful behaviour, there is clearly a need to have a serious talk with myself. Is my bad-tempered behaviour and irritability with my boss, colleagues and especially Sean making the slightest difference to sorting the issues out? Obviously the answer is no. They are just adding to my current difficulties. It is time to cut out the wine and slow down on the roads. And as for my current task, it's time to get cracking with it.'

Let's discover what actually happens when Zoe decides, following this pragmatic analysis of her new work situation, to put the above into action.

She begins the difficult task of trying to change her natural tendency to become irritable with colleagues and especially with Sean, often biting her tongue when she wants to lash out verbally. Sean suggests that she adopts a five-minute exercise and withdraws for a short period if she finds herself becoming irritable. She has to take a lot of short coffee and toilet breaks over the weeks that follow! It takes several months to gradually change her behaviour, but her hard work rapidly bears fruit, both at home and at work. She now no longer demands that everyone around her changes, but focuses instead on what she can do to sort out issues herself. She also disciplines herself to obey speed limits and seriously reduce her wine intake to weekends and small amounts.

Following a chat with Sean, their relationship now better than ever, she decides to visit head office and has some difficult conversations with senior management. They are reluctant to interfere in a local situation but do offer the choice of moving to a different department. Having weighed up all of the options, including researching the suggested department, Zoe decides to choose an alternative route. She contacts a close friend, working in a different company, and arranges a job interview with this group. She is successful and now finds herself working with a new team and a female boss, with whom she clicks immediately. She is careful, however, following her pragmatic analysis, to reassure her previous boss and colleagues that she is making the move for career reasons. She thus leaves her previous company on good terms.

Zoe has through this whole process learned some important lessons about herself and indeed about life. Life is full of disturbance and discomfort. People and situations don't change just because she would like this to happen. It is up to her and her alone to make the relevant changes in life, if she is unhappy or frustrated with something. She begins to put these insights into practice and discovers that her life is running much more smoothly than before. Life will, of course, fire some new change broadsides at her, but she is now armed with a pragmatic blueprint to resolve such situations.

The Baby Question

Let's now meet Paul, who is grappling with another common modern challenge. His partner, in her late thirties, decides that she would like to have another baby, a decision with which Paul fundamentally disagrees. This can be a regular source of conflict between couples. How many can relate to this dilemma? To have or not to have another baby? One could ask, 'Is there ever a right time to have a baby?' as life is fraught with so many potential reasons to delay such a decision. It can be a difficult question to answer, especially for many couples in their late thirties or early forties.

Sometimes there may be one or several children already present, but one partner pines to have another, to the dismay of the other. A significant issue can also develop when there is an understood, if sometimes unexpressed, agreement by the couple that there will be no children in a relationship and one partner then changes their mind on the issue. It is common, in both of these situations, for one or other party to become emotionally distressed, often with significant consequences. Paul falls into the first group. Let's see what happens when his wife Sara begins to pine for a further addition to their family unit.

Paul's Story

Paul, a forty-two-year-old self-employed businessman, has been married for seven years to Sara, who works as a receptionist in a local hotel. They have two children, Jack aged six and Mercy aged four, with both parents now really enjoying spending time with them.

Paul's business is getting increasingly busy and he has a staff of ten. Orders are piling in. Both customers and staff like him, even if he has the reputation of losing his cool if things are not going smoothly at work. He has always been someone who wants jobs done 'yesterday'. His team has learned to tiptoe around him if all is not going well. Overall, however, he manages his business life well, while trying to be available as much as possible to help Sara, who in turn has moved to part-time employment, to spend more time with the kids. All is well in their world.

Like many women who reach their late thirties, Sara, who has turned thirty-nine, begins to long for a further addition to their brood. The desire to have another child becomes increasingly consuming. She gently introduces the subject, but to her disappointment Paul reacts negatively. He becomes increasingly frustrated with her constant attempts to change his mind. Why, having working so hard to get to this point, would they mess it all up now? Was Sara not happy enough with their two lovely children? How would they cope with the major changes such a decision would introduce into their lives? Wouldn't another child just place enormous pressure on both of them, as individuals and as a couple? Has she forgotten how difficult the first few years following the arrival of Jack and Mercy were? Does she really want to return to that place again, just as all is going well in their lives?

Sara finds herself increasingly conflicted. She accepts that Paul is struggling with her wish to have another child. Yet her desire to have one final child becomes increasingly strong, especially when Jenny, one of her closest friends, has her third child at forty and is ecstatic. She continues to gently bring up the subject. Paul's frustration levels build up more. He becomes increasingly irritable and short with both her and the kids. At work, the staff notice the change. He becomes harder to work for, losing his rag with increasing frequency. The business suffers. Sara withdraws more in their relationship, feeling hurt that Paul is treating her the way he is. This increases his frustration further. He becomes more boorish on the road and hits the whiskey more. His life is slowly imploding. Finally, even Paul realizes that something will have to change. Things cannot go on as they are, or their relationship is heading for the rocks. Following a chat with his mum, a wise woman, he agrees to attend a therapist to thrash out the issues.

Now let's see what happens when Paul, on the advice of his therapist, applies the pragmatic blueprint to his current situation. Let's discover how he gradually rationalizes the situation, which is creating so much distress for himself and those he loves.

This is Paul's blueprint:

1. **How is this situation making me feel?**

   'Sara's desire to try for another child is making me feel extremely frustrated.'

2. **What is it about this situation that is causing me to feel this way?**

   'I am frustrated as I am being asked to accept a complete change in our current lives. Sara would love another baby but, if I am honest, I am struggling to accept the hassle that this will create. Why won't she listen to my sound advice and take heed of it? Can't she recognize the hard work involved in getting the two kids we already have to their current stage? Isn't now the time to relax and enjoy them? Can she not see that it will also create more pressure on me, just as the business is growing? If Sara would leave things as they are, all would be well.'

3. **What in my thinking is preventing me from dealing with this situation?**

   'I am demanding that I should not have to put up with the discomfort which the arrival of a new baby into the house will inevitably introduce. I am also demanding that Sara should see things as I see them, take my advice and decide not to travel down this road.'

4. **What in my behaviour is preventing me from dealing with this situation?**

    'In terms of my behaviour, I know that I am being irritable and bad-tempered with everyone, especially with Sara and the kids. I am also bad-tempered at work with customers and staff, which is not good for business. I am being ill-mannered on the road and drinking too much, neither of which is assisting matters.'

5. **How can I short-circuit my thinking and behavioural blocks to deal more effectively with this situation?**

    'I need to rethink some of my demands which on reflection seem unreasonable. I am refusing to accept that this decision is really important for Sara, irrespective of my opinions on the subject. It is completely understandable that Sara would desire to have a final child. If I love her as I do, I need to get off my self-centred perch and place myself in her shoes and try to understand where she is coming from. Is not our relationship and the love between us more important than any discomfort a new baby might bring?

    'I have to accept that discomfort is a part of life, so I cannot dodge it. Would it not be better, therefore, to accept the short-term discomfort and hassle that a further arrival might bring, for the long-term gain of seeing Sara happy and fulfilled in her life and not having to experience future long-term regrets?

    'A new arrival might also turn out to be a real blessing for the whole family unit, enriching it further. Not to mention the excitement that Jack and Mercy will experience at the arrival of a new sister or brother!

'In relation to my business, which is more important, making more money, or having a peaceful, warm, happy home life? I am good at what I do and well able to balance these two objectives. I just have to think about it differently.

'In relation to my unhelpful behaviour, it is clear what I have to do. I have to challenge my instinctive tendency to become irritable and bad-tempered with those around me if I am not getting my own way. I can see the ill effects of this on Sara and the two kids, not to mention at work! This change in my behaviour will have to extend to whiskey and my manners on the road, both of which I now accept are becoming a problem.

'Mostly, I have to sit down with Sara and have a good, frank conversation, reassuring her that I fully support her if she chooses to go down this road. I also need to apologize for my behaviour to date and promise to make things up to her, Jack and Mercy.

'I also need to re-engage with staff and customers at work and get us back to where we were. This will require a major change for one person in particular, namely me!'

Let's discover what actually happens when Paul decides, following this pragmatic analysis, to put the above ideas into action.

He begins with an emotional conversation with Sara. He apologizes for his behaviour to date, reassuring her that he is now fully on board with whatever decision she makes. Sara in turn empathizes with his concerns. They then thrash out all of the issues which could arise. She makes it clear, for example, that she is unwilling to go down the IVF route if she is unable to conceive naturally. If the latter does not occur within a year, she is happy to cease travelling down this road. Paul finds this extremely reassuring. They also explore the possibility that if a new baby were to arrive, Sara might give up her part-time work for a period of time to look after their children. Paul reassures her that his business is going well, so this would not be an issue financially. By the end of this conversation, both are fully on board with the decision to go ahead and try for a third child.

Paul, with Sara's assistance and that of his therapist, begins to challenge his behaviour both at work and at home. His therapist suggests that he withdraws for five minutes in such situations, if he senses he is going to blow a gasket. He finds this advice extremely helpful. He also learns to sit on himself when others are not seeing matters his way. Slowly but surely over the next six months, Paul finds himself becoming calmer and more tolerant. This has a positive effect at work and at home. His business begins to thrive as a consequence. He still loses it from time to time, as he is human like the rest of us, but now recognizes when this happens and quickly apologizes if appropriate. He understands that it is up to him to act if matters are not going according to plan, rather than trying to impose his view of the world on others, or expecting everyone else to change rather than himself.

Six months later, Sara, to the joy of both, conceives and subsequently delivers a healthy boy. Paul is overjoyed with the new arrival, John, who turns out to be a real character. Those around him suggest he is a cut-down version of Paul himself. Sara gives up her part-time job to concentrate on looking after their three children. Contrary to Paul's initial concerns, baby John is rapidly absorbed into their lives and it soon seems as if he has always been there. Paul and Sara, despite all of the normal pressures which arrive with a new baby, cope well and become even closer. Paul's new pragmatic approach to life and change has borne much new fruit!

PART FOUR

DEPRESSION

7. Why Change Can Make You Feel Depressed

There will be occasions in life when periods of change may lead to you feeling emotionally depressed. Perhaps you can relate to this emotional response when experiencing such periods. We are not discussing depression here as a clinical condition. Rather, we are discussing the unhealthy negative emotion of depression, with a little 'd', which most of us are familiar with. It is often described as 'feeling down' or 'going through a bout of the blues'.

But why does change make us feel emotionally depressed, and why do some of us experience this emotion more than others at such times? The answer lies in self-rating, something which many of us are unfortunately well acquainted with!

The World of Self-rating

Underlying the emotion of depression is the belief that you as a human being can be rated or measured or judged as a person, and that this personal rating can, on occasion, be pretty damning. This tendency to self-rate comes from the irrational belief that you must accept your own negative assessment of your worth or value as a human being. This form of negative self-rating is extremely prevalent in anxiety and depression, especially the latter.

In this scenario, it is easy to fall into the trap of defining yourself in some absolute terms as 'weak', 'worthless', 'a failure' and so on. You may notice how often you do just that when something in your life changes for the worse, often as a result of some actions you may have taken. You could, for example, fail an exam or job interview, and mercilessly self-flagellate yourself with such terms. The more you negatively self-rate in this manner, the more emotionally depressed you will feel.

This tendency to self-rate is being fed by the world you inhabit. Society is comfortable with the world of judgement and rating. Social media is built on this platform. It is a short step from this to believing that you as a human being can be rated by yourself or others.

On delving deeper into this tendency to self-rate, it becomes increasingly clear that you may be falling into the trap of merging who you are as a person with your behaviour or actions (including your skills and talents). Social media has really strengthened this connection. But even in the absence of this medium, many of us are already expert at doing just that.

If you can relate to this, notice how easy it is to travel up and down what we call the Rating Scale. Suppose I asked you to rate yourself as a person between one and a hundred, with one being low and a hundred being high. Most of us will give a figure between fifty and seventy or occasionally higher. A smaller number may rate themselves quite low, perhaps at twenty, as they may believe that that is 'all they are worth'. If I then asked you to rate yourself if successful at an exam or job interview, the results can be interesting. What was your response? The majority will immediately raise their rating to eighty or more. How about if I asked you then to rate yourself if unsuccessful at either? The majority will commonly drop their rating to lower levels, maybe thirty or forty. Did you do the same? If the answer to this is yes, you are, like the rest of us, playing the rating game. In this game, you rate yourself highly when things are going well and low if not!

Not a great recipe for emotional stability as you may discover your emotions, especially anxiety and depression, going up and down depending on what happens to you.

What you are doing, of course, is 'merging' who you are as a person with the success or failure of your actions or behaviour. Since the latter are inherently unstable, you may react to negative changes in your life by 'self-downing'. This allows your internal or pathological critic (PC) to swing into action. This is the voice in your head, shaped by your upbringing and events in your adult life, which tends to berate you intensely if things are not going well. This voice encourages you to describe yourself as 'a failure' or 'useless' or 'worthless' and so on.

If you can recognize this pattern and you notice that this is often your go-to response to some negative change in your life, such as failing to get that job you really wanted, for example, then you are playing the rating game. This is unfortunately a game which nobody wins!

The pragmatic approach to the world of self-rating is to challenge whether human beings are like objects or works of art which can be assessed and rated, or bought and sold. The answer is clearly no, so why continue with this destructive tendency? It would also challenge you to accept that your actions and behaviours are definitely open to rating or assessment. In this scenario, you have a duty and responsibility to make sure such actions are appropriate and not, for example, hurting other people.

Pragmatism would encourage you especially to develop the art of unconditional self-acceptance, a concept which I have discussed in detail in previous books. This is where you learn to love and accept yourself for the beautiful and unique human being that you are but also take responsibility for your actions or behaviour. It would also challenge the language of the PC as described above. Can a human being be a failure, for example, or is it preferable to describe something you have tried to do (such as a job interview or exam) which has failed? If the latter, the pragmatist would counsel: get up and try again! I have often described unconditional self-acceptance as the ultimate emotional resilience skill and the bedrock of good mental health.

The Role of Your Behaviour

How you respond behaviourally when change makes you depressed can also add to your problems. There are many destructive behaviours which you may recognize in yourself. These are all created as a response to feeling emotionally down, which in turn is triggered by the above instinctive tendency to self-rate when life is going pear-shaped, as it is wont to do.

Many of these behavioural patterns relate to your lifestyle. You may notice how you withdraw socially and emotionally from others, often spending increasing time on your own, perhaps in your bedroom. You may eat poorly or drink more than usual. You may notice how your exercise regimes fall away and you lose interest in normal daily life. Usually and thankfully, these behavioural patterns are of short duration and improve when your mood lifts. You may also notice at such times how you seek out only the negative, especially in relation to social media and news outlets.

The pragmatic view of such behaviour is to challenge whether such actions are assisting you to challenge your self-rating or indeed lift your mood. Clearly, they are usually having an opposite effect. The message is obvious. You have to challenge such behaviours, even if it is difficult.

The really positive news is that you can learn new pragmatic ways of thinking and behaviour to manage this emotion, if it is your natural 'go-to' place, when some negative change in your life occurs. Let's explore how this would work in practice.

8. How to Manage Your 'Change' Depression

The Pragmatic Approach to Depression

In the previous chapter, we discussed how, if your normal response to change is depression, you are most likely playing the rating game. Depending on whether you are successful or not in your actions, talents, skills or behaviours, you judge or measure yourself up or down, and how destructive that can be to your mental health.

The pragmatic reality, of course, is that nobody can actually measure or judge or rate another human being as a person, as each one of us is special and unique. If you do not believe me, put your children or brothers and sisters or parents or good friends together on a couch and rate one over the other. Not so easy to do this in practice, is it? Your natural response to rating your children, for example, will be 'How can I do this, as Vanessa is so different from William?' And you are so right in this assessment. We are all just too unique and special.

But you can definitely rate or measure or judge the effectiveness of your actions or behaviours and others are entitled to do so as well. What you are not advised to do, however, is base your assessment of yourself as a person, as a special, unique human being, on how such actions or behaviours turn out. Life is extremely fickle. Sometimes you will notch up a 'win' in such situations, but more often may experience a 'loss'. Neither will define who you are as a person.

Pragmatism would encourage you to develop instead the art of unconditional self-acceptance. This is where you learn to love and accept yourself for the beautiful and unique human being you are, but take responsibility for your actions or behaviour. It would also counsel you to challenge and change many of the unhelpful behaviours such as self-isolation which simply strengthen your feelings of depression.

But how can you apply the above pragmatic conclusions to periods of change in your life? The answer lies in applying the five-question pragmatic blueprint, outlined in earlier chapters, to analyse such periods.

Let's see how this would work by meeting Jonathan, who is encountering a period of upheaval that is common in the lives of many young people, namely the struggle to gain sufficient points in state exams to enter a desired college course. Perhaps you, too, can see yourself in his story.

Jonathan's Story

Jonathan is an eighteen-year-old student who is desperate to get enough points to qualify for a particular college course, but misses out by five points and becomes emotionally depressed. To Jonathan, it is a disaster. For years, he has judged himself based on his academic achievements. His whole sense of himself and what others (in his mind) think of him depends on his success or failure in this key area of his life.

This is compounded by his obsession with how others view him on social media.

Clearly Jonathan is falling into the trap of playing the rating game. He is now faced with a period of change in his life, where he has to adapt and think outside the box. He is merging who he is with how successful or not he is academically. This combination of feeling emotionally depressed secondary to his destructive self-downing, and some unhelpful behaviours, are preventing him from managing this period of stressful change.

His story is replicated over and over, year after year, as countless students in schools and colleges fall into the same emotional, thinking and behavioural errors, often suffering significant emotional distress as a consequence.

Let's see how Jonathan, by applying our five-question pragmatic blueprint on paper, discovers a new path out of his difficulties.

Here is Jonathan's blueprint:

1. **How is this situation making me feel?**
   'My emotion is depression.'

2. **What is it about this situation that is causing me to feel this way?**
   'I have failed in my task of achieving sufficient points to get in to my course, so I now believe that I am a failure. I also see myself as useless.'

3. **What in my thinking is preventing me from dealing with this situation?**
   'Because I have failed to get into the only course I was interested in doing, I am a failure and useless.'

4. **What in my behaviour is preventing me from dealing with this situation?**

   'I am withdrawing from all my friends and family, have lost interest in food, am binge-drinking if I do go out and struggling to seek out any other avenues to get where I want.'

5. **How can I short-circuit my thinking and behavioural blocks to deal more effectively with this situation?**

   'I need to stop rating myself so harshly as useless and a failure and need to accept myself just for being myself, but accept responsibility for my behaviour.

   'In relation to my behaviour, I need to socialize more, cease my alcohol binges and begin to seek out other alternatives (such as repeating exams, doing courses that would feed into the course I want to do, etc.) to get to where I want to go.'

The good news is that Jonathan, as a result of this analysis, makes some key decisions. He decides to repeat his exams, but also to take on some part-time work in the hospitality sector at the same time. This teaches him many life skills which he otherwise would have missed out on. He learns a lot about life itself in the process. Life is not perfect and neither is he. Failure is a normal part of life, it is the 'trying again' part that really matters. Most of all, he learns to accept that he is just a normal bloke like the rest of humanity, with strengths and weaknesses, and to be comfortable with who he is and cease trying to be someone he is not.

The following year, Jonathan is successful in his exams and begins the course of his dreams as a more rounded, emotionally mature student. It is his perseverance combined with unconditional self-acceptance, and not his academic brilliance, which wins the day!

Now let's meet Jim, Pauline and Philip, each of whom is undergoing a difficult transitional period of change in their lives and reacting with feelings of depression. We will discover, with the assistance of our pragmatic blueprint, how they, too, discover new solutions to their situations.

Loss of Job/Retirement

We begin by visiting with Jim, who is experiencing a common cause of change leading to emotional distress, namely retirement. For many of us, retirement is a period to look forward to. An opportunity to let go of strict structures, rigid deadlines and, on occasion, long commutes. A period bristling with new opportunities to engage in different hobbies and activities. The closing of one chapter in our life and the opening of a new one.

For some, however, and Jim belongs to this group, retirement can be one of the most challenging periods of our adult life. So much of our lives are taken up by the domain of work, for better or for worse. Our social world is also commonly connected with work colleagues or mates. Much of the structure of our days and weeks is taken up with the routines of the normal working day.

When we find ourselves, as a result of retirement, suddenly bereft of these structures, routines and social connections, it is easy to become lost, to lose our sense of purpose and meaning. It is a short step from this, as Jim discovers, to becoming emotionally depressed. Let's explore just how he comes to terms with this major period of change in his life. There will be many, many readers who will empathize with his story!

Jim's Story

Jim, who has just turned sixty-five, has been happily married to Jenifer for thirty-five years. They have two adult children, Maura, who resides permanently with her partner in Australia, and Matthew, living and working in Belgium. Jim and Jenifer have always enjoyed a great relationship. This is about to come under significant pressure.

Jim has worked all of his life as a community postman and is widely known and liked within his local community. He has an organized structure and routine to his day. Despite occasional weather challenges, Jim lives for his work. He particularly enjoys the social aspect of being a postman. Those regular chats with the public, and the camaraderie with colleagues. Each Christmas, he is showered with gifts from appreciative customers.

As he comes closer to the date of his retirement, former colleagues who have travelled down this road ahead of him warn him about how much his life will change. They suggest taking some pre-retirement courses to prepare him. But Jim, always the optimistic extrovert, dismisses such suggestions. He has always coped with periods of change and this will be no different.

Eventually retirement arrives. Jim enjoys a great send-off and is especially chuffed with his retirement present, a beautiful watch, which he greatly treasures.

Then reality strikes home, as Jim finds the first few weeks following his retirement especially challenging. He has always been an early riser, but now struggles with the cold reality that there is no longer any reason to continue this pattern of a lifetime. He fixes everything around the house, but rapidly runs out of tasks. He finds himself with large swathes of time and is at a loss as to how best to use them. He struggles to create any kind of structure or routine in his new life. He feels like a rudderless ship, adrift on the high seas. He has never been interested in reading or music. He watches TV or listens to the radio aimlessly, without seeing or hearing much of what is being said.

What he misses most are those daily social conversations with customers and colleagues. He is not a man for the pub or for sport and lacks any real hobbies.

He and Jenifer have travelled abroad, but Jim has never really enjoyed the experience. His whole life has revolved around work. He constantly reflects on how quickly one can become an unimportant and insignificant player in other people's lives. Someone else is now performing what had been his job. He is now forgotten, insignificant, of little value to himself or others. He remembers something that Jenifer once revealed to him whilst going through the horrors of the menopause. How she had felt 'invisible'. Jim had never really understood what his wife was describing until now. This is exactly how he feels, invisible and useless!

Increasingly he ruminates as to how irrelevant he and his life have become. He avoids the very people whom he has served for so long. He believes that others will now see him, as he sees himself, as useless, no longer of use to them or indeed himself. Someone to say a polite hello to and move on. Much of this is emanating from his emotional mind, of course, but Jim struggles to see this at the time. He stays increasingly at home, even hitting the bottle of whiskey in the evening, just feeling increasingly isolated and depressed.

For Jenifer, too, Jim's retirement becomes increasingly problematic. It feels to her as if a bombshell has dropped into their previously happy, organized, structured life that both had enjoyed for over thirty years. She is not used to having Jim around the place, finding his attempts at helping with routine domestic chores more of a hindrance than a help. He is better taking care of the garden and sheds or sorting out their finances. She really misses having her two children around, and especially their grandchildren. The weekly online chats are great but can't replace those real-life, one-to-one, face-to-face conversations.

She is also becoming increasingly worried about Jim, whom she loves dearly, even if he is now constantly under her feet domestically. She can see that he is missing the routines and social nourishment which his job provided but is at her wits' end as to how best to assist him. Jim is not renowned for taking advice at the best of times and this is no different. He is clearly down at times and she notes his increasing attachment to whiskey, something foreign to him. She seeks advice from her children and sister, with the latter having experienced a similar situation several years previously.

Thankfully, before Jim's situation deteriorates further, a colleague, Mark, who retired several years previously, comes to see him, and they have a good chat. Mark suggests a serious rethink about Jim's current situation and how he is approaching it, sharing with him some of his own experiences. Mark is a pragmatist, a problem solver.

Now let's see what happens when Jim, at Mark's suggestion, applies our pragmatic blueprint to the issues arising from his retirement.

Here are Jim's conclusions:

1. **How is this situation making me feel?**

    'My recent retirement has resulted in me becoming emotionally depressed.'

2. **What is it about this situation that is causing me to feel this way?**

    'I am feeling depressed as my retirement has altered or changed everything about my previous life. I no longer believe I am useful or of value, and I feel simply invisible. I feel trapped, my normal routines and structures now gone. I struggle to fill my days with anything meaningful. I am driving Jenifer crazy, under her feet all the time, making me believe I am even more useless. I miss the social contacts that I enjoyed with customers and colleagues. I now believe that I am of no interest or value to them as I am no longer performing the job I love. I now understand that I had become my job! Without it, I am nothing!'

3. **What in my thinking is preventing me from dealing with this situation?**

    'I am falling into the trap of believing that because my job and everything which goes with it is gone, I am useless, of little value or worth to myself or others, invisible. Even writing this down is shocking. Do I really believe this about myself?'

4. **What in my behaviour is preventing me from dealing with this situation?**

    'In terms of my behaviour, I know that I am moody and difficult to live with. I can feel myself withdrawing from life and know that this is not healthy, neither good for me nor for Jenifer. I am sensible enough to see that the whiskey is not helping, just making me feel more depressed the following day. Nor are my decisions to cease exercising and to avoid meeting customers or the general public assisting in sorting all of this out.'

5. **How can I short-circuit my thinking and behavioural blocks to deal more effectively with this situation?**

'In relation to my distorted thinking, I need to seriously relook at how I am describing myself as a person. Can a human being be seriously rated or judged as invisible or useless in real life? Maybe it's time to challenge these voices in my head, as Mark suggests. Mark also shared with me a concept, picked up in his local Men's Shed, which I really liked, namely that we must learn to unconditionally love and accept ourselves for the special human beings we are. I love this idea as it frees me up to be who I really am. Mark himself commented to me how this had assisted him in dealing with similar negative thoughts following his retirement. I am going to fully embrace this idea! That human beings cannot be simply defined as useless or worthless as these are simply tags or labels, signifying little. It will be tough, but I have to challenge these negative thoughts, as they are just bringing me down. Mark makes one other important point, namely that retirement becomes what you decide it to be. If you choose to look at it as being trapped, with no place to go, then you will continue to feel depressed. If, on the other hand, you redefine it as an opportunity, then a whole new world opens up. I like this idea, too.

Maybe it is time for a new approach and I was never one to shirk a challenge.

'In terms of behaviour, there is much to do. I am going to put into practice another of Mark's suggestions, which is to establish a new organized daily structure. Go to bed and get up at the same time. Exercise more and if you do meet someone, stop and chat about what is going on in their lives and not mine. Cease the whiskey. Get out of Jenifer's hair. Join some community groups. Mark has offered to assist me in joining our local Men's Shed. This is a place where men come together to make useful creations for the community, but also to chat and share stories about their mental-wellbeing difficulties. Mark assures me that there are many men of my age experiencing similar issues, who find the Shed life-saving. He also suggests joining the local Tidy Towns group and offering my services for the Meals on Wheels group, who deliver meals to senior infirm or housebound citizens. I like the sound of both of these. Mark has also offered to introduce me to his pitch-and-putt mates, which sounds like great fun. The best advice Mark gave me, however, was to find tasks that give me meaning, as without this it is hard to keep on living. I need to replace the meaning which my job once brought me with community activities, especially helping those more vulnerable. As he good-humouredly notes: "If you want to be truly miserable, just give yourself your total undivided attention!" He is right, it is time to stop feeling sorry for myself, give myself a good kick in the backside, and get out there and help others who may be less fortunate.'

Let's now find out what actually happens when Jim decides, following this pragmatic analysis and with Mark's assistance, to put the above into action.

He begins at the root of the problem, his belief that following his retirement from the job he so loved, he is no longer useful or of value to himself or anyone else. On Mark's suggestion, he writes down what his emotional mind is telling him and then challenges it on paper. He has always been a man of logic, so rapidly accepts just how illogical these self-descriptions are. He works hard at developing unconditional self-acceptance. With Jenifer's assistance and encouragement, he develops a more realistic, pragmatic view of himself as a person and how to focus more on his behaviour. He learns to rethink many of his false opinions about retirement. Is it not simply an opportunity, as Mark has suggested, to become involved in other areas of community life, ignored by him to date? He begins to view retirement from a completely different perspective, and this makes all the difference.

He changes many of his unhealthy lifestyle habits. Out go the whiskey and self-isolation. In come a proper sleep, exercise and dietary regime, along with a more structured approach to his days. His first objective is to emerge from under poor Jenifer's feet. With Mark, he attends his local Men's Shed and discovers a second home. There he finds a group of men experiencing similar difficulties, some following retirement and others dealing with unemployment. They meet regularly, to complete different projects to help their community. But what Jim comes to value most are the conversations between them. Each man sharing their particular story or journey, noting how friendship and comradeship is keeping them bonded together.

He also becomes active in other community activities. He enjoys delivering Meals on Wheels to senior and vulnerable citizens who are isolated and frequently lonely. Many of them remember him fondly from his postman days, and soon he has a new social group to chat to each day. He also joins the Tidy Towns committee, which keeps him extremely busy. Mark also drags him out to play pitch and putt. Soon he grows to love the game, making many new friends in the process.

Within six months, Jenifer is (happily) used to Jim being constantly busy with all of these activities. She is delighted to see him back to his old self, smiling and laughing, full of chat and stories about his many and varied experiences. As he comments to Mark a year later, retirement from his old job has now become a distant memory, a chapter in the book of his life that he has closed. He has learned pragmatically how to embrace change. That has made all of the difference!

Becoming a New Parent

Now let's meet Pauline, about to experience another common, often stressful, period of change, namely the arrival home of a first child. In our fast-moving, technological world, many couples are choosing, for career and other reasons, to start their families later, often in their mid- to late-thirties. While this event brings with it emotions of great joy and happiness, the first six to twelve months especially can also be enormously stressful, especially for the mother. While the father in these situations will also experience significant stress and even occasionally bouts of low mood, it is frequently the mother who bears the brunt of the psychological impact of this period of change. It is common, as happens with Pauline, for many mothers to experience the emotion of depression. Others may become so overwhelmed by the stress and psychological impact of the arrival of the new baby that it triggers a full-blown bout of postnatal depression, or PND.

This is unsurprising, as this is a period where, as a new mum, change enters your life with a vengeance. It begins with the exhaustion of the last few weeks of pregnancy. It continues with the trauma of the delivery, with many women feeling as if their body has been pulled asunder. It continues, following the initial high of seeing and holding your new baby, with the exhaustion of trying to recover from the trauma of the childbirth, while up, day and night, feeding your baby. All of the time trying to keep up an appearance for your partner, family and friends that you are coping wonderfully!

Then you arrive home to face the reality that you and your partner are now on your own with this little bundle, uncertain every step of the way as to what or what not to do to ensure your baby stays healthy and well. Even experienced midwives bringing home their baby for the first time admit to feeling stressed and anxious at this point. If you are fortunate enough to have a mother or sibling close by, this can lighten the load. But nowadays many couples live far away from family and community supports. You are often on your own and feeling lost. While increasingly fathers may take a week or two off to assist when the baby arrives, from then on the buck stops literally with you, the mum!

There are few new mothers who cannot relate to what happens next. You find yourself increasingly fatigued from lack of sleep and the relentless cycles of feeding and changing routines, continuing day and night, week after week, month after month. Your partner may want to assist with night feeds, but this may not be that easy to organize with breastfeeding on demand. You begin to crave sleep above all else. You may still be trying to come to terms with the assault on your body from the labour itself, or perhaps you are coping with a healing episiotomy wound or bleeding. You may find yourself losing interest in your appearance due to exhaustion from this relentless routine. Meanwhile you still try to present the best picture possible to your partner, family and friends.

Above all, you want to hide from them how much you are really struggling. You may find yourself also falling into the fatal trap of assuming that other women are coping much better than you, especially with social-media platforms showing them looking fantastic and seemingly coping so well. You may find yourself wondering 'What is wrong with me, why am I not coping as well as other women are? Why is this whole period, which I so looked forward to, turning into a bit of a nightmare?'

And then comes the screaming, the dreaded three-month colic. Your previously content baby begins to scream uncontrollably, often beginning in the evenings from six to ten, for hours without end, no matter what you or your partner do. Eventually and thankfully, as if by magic, the screaming usually stops after three months and you begin at last to feel as if you are getting on top of things.

This is often followed, however, by the baby now waking up at night with red cheeks, once again howling, as the whole process of teething begins. More sleepless nights, more exhaustion!

You may also find that this period of change brings with it intense loneliness. You may find yourself cut off from normal social relationships and friendships. You may find yourself 'brain-dead' from lack of sleep, exhaustion, the constant grind of looking after your baby whilst completing normal household chores, even if these tasks are divided between you as a couple.

And as for the strain on your relationship, nothing could have prepared you for it. It is hard to go from a full-on hectic personal and social life as a couple to an almost non-existent one. You may even feel yourself losing interest in your looks and appearance.

And as for intimacy! Sleep is all you really crave. Some couples describe the first six to twelve months following the arrival of a new baby into their relationship as 'Armageddon'. It is easy to see why!

What was an organized, busy, working, personal and social life is now reduced to an hour by hour, day by day, week by week ongoing struggle for survival, with everything you thought certain now blown out the window.

Many mums comment on how they cope better with subsequent babies, as they know what to expect and are better prepared. It is still challenging for many couples to survive these periods. It is tough! Anyone who tells you otherwise has either never experienced the situation, has reared an incredibly well-behaved baby or is simply not admitting to the truth, with the latter being the most common.

Difficulties arise, however, when you begin to feel emotionally down or depressed, from assuming that there must be something wrong with you in that you are not coping as well as you believe other women are. There is little doubt that the celebrity social-media pictures and videos (discussed above) of the 'perfect mum' will not assist you here. For such pictures do not represent real life. Behind these pictures usually lies a retinue of staff who are looking after the baby in question. But you may also be looking at normal social-media sites or hearing stories where colleagues or friends or siblings 'seem' to be coping so much better than you. This can lead you to erroneously believe that you are a failure, with depression being the emotion beckoning in such situations. This is what happens to Pauline. Let's see how her story unfolds.

Pauline's Story
Pauline is thirty-seven and lives with her partner Val, who works as a quantity surveyor for a large construction

company. Having lived together for four years, and following several miscarriages and rounds of IVF, to the great joy of all concerned, Pauline delivers a healthy baby boy, Luke. She has experienced a difficult pregnancy, spending the last few weeks in hospital with high blood pressure or pre-eclampsia. Following a long and difficult labour and delivery, she is physically and mentally drained. Initially this is forgotten, as both she and Val are overjoyed with the arrival of this little bundle into their lives, made all the sweeter following her difficulties with miscarriages and IVF.

Pauline, following this short period of sheer joy, finds herself feeling both exhausted and low in mood, but copes with both while still in hospital. But on arrival home with Luke, the reality of how much their lives are about to change dawns on both, especially Pauline. Val is around for the first ten days but subsequently she finds herself increasingly alone during the daytime, as family and in-laws live some distance away at the other end of the country. To all intents and purposes, she is on her own.

Thus begins a really difficult time for Pauline and her partner. Her sleep patterns become completely disrupted as she is breastfeeding on demand. Within weeks, she becomes increasingly exhausted. Val does his best to assist her in any way he can, but despite this it is a struggle. Luke is also slow to gain weight as Pauline experiences significant difficulties with breastfeeding. The public-health nurse becomes concerned about this and discusses the possibility of switching to bottle-feeding if this continues. Pauline has always assumed that she would cope well with her new baby. Has she not been dreaming of this moment for years? How could she let her baby down so badly?

The following weeks and months become a nightmare for Pauline and Val. Luke begins to howl non-stop, every evening from six weeks onwards. Initially she and Val panic, assuming that there must be something seriously wrong with Luke. Thankfully a chat with their family doctor provides an explanation, if not necessarily a respite. Luke is suffering from three-month colic. Knowing what it is, however, doesn't make it any less difficult to cope with. They take turns in walking up and down for hours with their screaming baby, but nothing seems to work. Pauline finds herself increasingly breaking down into tears with frustration and exhaustion. Nobody has prepared her for this. Just when she feels as if she is going to have a complete breakdown, at around three months Luke suddenly stops crying.

She also continues to have difficulties with Luke struggling to gain weight. Finally, and with assistance from her public-health nurse and family doctor, a decision is made to switch to bottle-feeding. This at least allows Val to assist with night feeds, enabling Pauline to get some sleep.

Then the teething process begins and their temporary calm is shattered. Luke once again starts to howl, presenting with red cheeks and drooling, all occurring primarily in the middle of the night. Both Val and Pauline are now struggling, with their sleep patterns constantly disrupted.

Pauline also finds it difficult to come to terms with other major changes brought on by the arrival of Luke. She especially misses her friends and work colleagues and the normal human interactions she has taken for granted up to this point in her life. There is simply no time to work on these, however. By the end of each day she is just wiped and ready for bed. She tries to keep in contact using social media, but this makes her feel worse, as everyone else seems to be coping better than she is. There is certainly no mention of colic or teething. What is she doing wrong? She also admits to Val how her brain has gone to mush. How is she ever going to return to work after six months? She is brain-dead.

At the same time, Pauline is experiencing intermittent periods of low mood, with Val wondering if she is developing postnatal depression. She has a good chat with her family doctor about this possibility. Her GP, who has small children herself, reassures her that what she is experiencing is normal. Although Pauline is experiencing drops in mood, these are not continuous. The more likely source of her symptoms lies with the stress of coping with her new baby and her chronic lack of sleep. The GP suggests more exercise, bringing the baby with her, and seeking out further assistance from family or friends.

But Pauline continues to struggle with her mood intermittently dropping. She is increasingly rating herself negatively as a failure and useless, adding to her emotion of depression. She pulls back more from both Val and Luke and even her appetite and weight are beginning to suffer. She resists going down the alcohol route, knowing where this might lead. She becomes obsessive about checking how other mothers are doing online and this makes her feel even more depressed.

Thankfully, before Pauline slips into a bout of PND, help arrives in the form of her mother, who has noted on Skype that her daughter is struggling and seems low in mood and so decides to visit for a few weeks. Pauline reveals all to her mum. She in turn shares with her daughter how she had undergone a similar experience with her first child. How she had experienced PND and the lessons she learned from this period. Her mum is also a complete pragmatist, so she encourages Pauline to go down this route. Her life is about to change for the better.

Let's see what happens when Pauline, with her mum's assistance, begins to apply our pragmatic blueprint to the issues arising from the arrival of her new baby.

Here are Pauline's findings and conclusions:

1. **How is this situation making me feel?**
   'Since the birth of Luke and the subsequent difficulties experienced, I have become emotionally depressed.'

2. **What is it about this situation that is causing me to feel this way?**
   'I am feeling depressed because I genuinely believe that I have been a complete failure as a mother and on occasion as a partner. I completely lack the skills to deal with Luke when he is distressed from colic and teething. I have failed in the most basic mothering skill of all, namely being able to breastfeed my own child. I feel depressed at finding myself "brain-dead" since Luke's arrival, as this makes me believe that I am of less value to him and to Val. I also feel abnormal in comparison to so many of my online "friends" who are coping so well with their first-born babies, despite having experienced similar challenges. So, what's wrong with me?'

3. **What in my thinking is preventing me from dealing with this situation?**
   'I can now identify how, as a result of the difficulties created by Luke's arrival and my struggle to deal with them, I now see myself as useless, a failure and abnormal.'

4. **What in my behaviour is preventing me from dealing with this situation?**

'In terms of my behaviour, I know that my gradual withdrawal from Val and Luke is not healthy for them or me. I have stopped my exercise and fitness regimes. I am not eating properly. I have also become obsessed with my social media and feeds, constantly comparing myself to others.'

5. **How can I short-circuit my thinking and behavioural blocks to deal more effectively with this situation?**

'In relation to my thinking, I can now see that I am being extremely self-deprecating and hard on myself. When I look at the language I am using about myself, written down in my own handwriting, it's pretty clear that these terms are vague, negative and extremely personal. Am I really useless, or a failure or abnormal? As my mum correctly points out, are these not simply describing my actions or skills, rather than me as a person?

'Is it not that my struggle to cope with my new baby lies at the heart of my current difficulties? Whilst I may be failing in some people's eyes to cope with Luke when he has colic or is teething, does that really mean that I am a failure as a person? Is this not just a vague form of self-rating, which means very little in practice? Maybe I am underestimating just how difficult it is to learn the ropes of how to look after a new baby. After all, there is no other way of learning how to do so, apart from experience, and perhaps simply trying and failing regularly. Is this not just life? I now realize from talking to Mum, who is an extremely competent person, that she too had a difficult time postnatally, even enduring a bout of postnatal depression, and she had more supports at the time than I have.

'Val, and my family and friends, do not see me as a failure or useless. So why am I applying these derogatory terms to myself? As Mum explains, it is the situation that is abnormal, not me! I now understand better that how I feel and the difficulties I have experienced during this period are universal. There are many other mums in the same boat as me, and they too are struggling. Is it just that some of them are putting on a public face that all is well, while underneath their lives remain as scattered as mine?

'It is also such a relief to learn from Mum that being "brain-dead" is normal during this period, with lack of sleep and the absence of normal life greatly contributing to this. Even more of a relief to hear that it gradually clears away over the first six to twelve months!

'Maybe I need to do as Mum has suggested and learn to accept myself unconditionally as a human being who is doing her best in very trying conditions. Even writing this down is making me feel much better about myself. I feel freer and am no longer experiencing the burden of expectations on my back. It doesn't mean, of course, that I can stop being responsible for my actions or behaviour or cease doing my best in every situation. I just need to be kinder to myself.

'In terms of my behaviour, I can now see how unhelpful some of my actions have been. I need to start taking better care of myself in terms of nutrition and exercise for starters. I have to do my best to get my life, including Luke, into a more organized structure and routine, with the assistance of Val, Mum and close friends, with whom I am now determined to share my trials.

'I also need to reach out to other mums in a similar situation and share experiences with them, as withdrawal and isolation are not helping my mood. Above all, I need to switch off my Instagram and Facebook feeds and cease torturing myself with false information as to how everyone else is seemingly coping so well.'

Let's now see what actually happens when Pauline decides, following this pragmatic analysis and with her mum's assistance, to put the above changes into action.

She begins by focusing more on herself, especially on her diet, exercise and self-care, and gradually feels better about herself. With the assistance of the public-health nurse, Pauline makes contact with several mother-and-baby groups who meet regularly. This turns out to be a real game-changer. As they share stories of their experiences of pregnancy, childbirth and especially the first six months postnatally, Pauline quickly realizes that almost all of them are in the same boat as her. She makes many new friends, and they link up regularly, even enjoying special film shows where mums and babies watch movies together. They also share parenting tips and techniques, many of which Pauline finds especially helpful.

The more she learns, the more she notices how her thinking is becoming increasingly realistic. She comes to an understanding that it is her emotional mind that is the source of her beliefs that she is a failure or abnormal. Many mums share their experiences of believing that they, too, were failures or worthless. Pauline works hard on trying to develop unconditional self-acceptance, sharing this concept with the other mums, to great effect. Her emotion of depression rapidly becomes a distant memory.

Bit by bit, Luke grows and life for Pauline and Val becomes easier. After six months, she returns to work part-time, and finds herself coping better than expected, with all the information she has acquired. By the end of the first year, her early postnatal difficulties are a distant memory. As she admits to her mum on the phone, they are now even considering the possibility of a further addition to their family.

Relationship Break-ups

In the last of our three cases, where change leads to the emotion of depression, we are going to visit with Philip, who is grappling with the harsh reality of a major relationship break-up. Human relationships by their nature are extremely complex. There are few areas of life, however, which can create as much emotional distress as the break-up of a personal relationship, especially where the couple have lived together for a considerable period. The changes that such a break-up can introduce into our lives are profound and can be a frequent cause of depression the emotion or, in extreme cases, even bouts of clinical depression.

Break-ups frequently occur at key transitional moments in our lives. It is common, for example, for young adults who have been together for several years as adolescents to separate around the age of twenty-one or so, with both sexes, especially girls, changing significantly around this age. It is also routine to see break-ups occurring in couples in their late twenties, who may have been living together for years. It can be especially problematic, for both men and women, if a break-up happens to couples in their late thirties or early forties, with the latter often experiencing additional worries about their fertility levels reducing with age.

Break-ups later in life can also present major challenges, when couples with children of varying ages decide to go their own ways. This can introduce a completely new set of life changes, which can threaten to overwhelm either party. This, as we shall see, is what happens to Philip. There is also an increasing trend for relationships to break up when couples are in their fifties or sixties. This, too, can present its own set of challenges in coping with the changes encountered in the lives of those affected.

There are two consistent threads present in most break-ups. The first is that the lives of both people are going to change, in some cases dramatically. The second is that this change is going to be associated with some significant emotions, often distressing ones. There is usually considerable sadness about the loss of the relationship, but also anxiety about the future, hurt about how it happens (which we will explore in subsequent chapters), anger, even guilt. One of the commonest emotional responses is depression, as Philip discovers. One might ask: why does a relationship break-up lead to one or other of those involved experiencing depression? The answer is simple. Relationship break-ups can trigger some intense negative self-criticism, whereby you see yourself as a failure or useless or of little value to yourself or others. This can lead to your internal critic ruminating constantly, berating you for being stupid, a failure, worthless, etc., which, as already discussed, drives the emotion of depression.

But it is also important to explore why break-ups cause so much change to our lives. If break-ups happen in our early to mid-twenties, these changes are often of less significance than for long-term relationships or partnerships that break up when the couple are in their forties, for example. In the case of the latter, there are usually major financial and social consequences when a couple or family unit splits, especially if children are involved.

Depending on the financial circumstances of the household, break-ups can cause difficulties for both parties, as sometimes properties have to be sold, arrangements for maintenance of children sorted out and so on. This can put great emotional strain on both parties, especially if confrontation is present.

The second major change relates to the loss on both sides of a wider social network of family and friends, which both routinely share. This can lead to symptoms of loneliness or increased isolation. Then there is the loss of the constant presence of children (in many cases), even if joint custody is agreed.

When break-ups occur in the twenties or early thirties, there are usually fewer financial issues unless children are involved. But the change to the social fabric of both lives can still be extensive, with loneliness becoming an issue for some, especially in the period after the split. Clearly in many cases the break-up is amicable, there are no children present and both sides are happy to move on to new pastures, but this can be more difficult for some than others. It can be challenging for both parties in a break-up, whatever the age at which it occurs, to adapt to the new situation in which they find themselves.

It is not just the emotional response to such changes that can create problems for us, however; it is also our behavioural responses to such emotions. In the case of depression, you may notice how you pull away from people, eat poorly, exercise less, cease taking care of your physical appearance, become more apathetic and sometimes take refuge in the bottle. None of these behaviours will assist you in dealing with the issues underlying the change.

If you are someone who has experienced or is going through such an experience, or have friends or family encountering a similar one, you may find Philip's story resonating with you.

Philip's Story

Philip is forty-nine and married to Olive. They have two sons, aged twelve and ten. He works as a middle manager in a medium-sized company, while Olive works as a dental nurse. They met when he was thirty-four and, for him, there was never going to be anyone else. For the first ten years of their marriage, life was good. Like all couples, they had their ups and downs, but their relationship in general was reasonably good. Over the next five years, however, things slowly unravelled.

Philip finds himself forced to travel as part of his job. Between financial pressures, commuting and the sheer effort of modern life, their relationship slowly disintegrates. Communication becomes increasingly fraught and intimacy gradually dries up. Rows flare up over smaller and smaller issues until they find themselves slowly drifting apart. Olive, for the sake of their children, chooses to remain in the relationship, but over time even this decision becomes problematic. Matters come to a head when she finds herself increasingly drawn, romantically, to a work colleague.

She comes clean with Philip, seeking a separation. In her mind, their marriage and relationship is over and she no longer has feelings for him. Philip is devastated but, following a long conversation, admits that their relationship is in deep trouble. He suggests counselling, but Olive feels it is too late for this step.

What follows for Philip is a nightmare period of change. While both agree to amicably separate and to engage a mediation service, nothing prepares him for the reality of their separation. They sell their property, pay off their mortgage, agree maintenance and go their separate ways. The children stay with Olive, with the amicable agreement that Philip will have regular access.

Olive by nature is more pragmatic and finds it easier to move on with her life.

Not so Philip, whose whole world is now turned upside down as he struggles to cope with the changes suddenly introduced into his life. The first major change is financial, as he discovers that renting a new apartment, paying maintenance and creating some form of new life for himself proves to be costly. He also finds his social world imploding as it had been primarily based on his relationship with Olive and her friends, family and in-laws. Now that is gone, he spends increasing time alone and lonely. He sees the boys regularly and they sometimes stay over, giving him a brief lift. When they return to their mum, however, he feels even more bereft. Matters are not helped when he hears that Olive is now dating her work colleague. Friends who have undergone similar experiences share with him how difficult coping with separation can be.

He feels constantly sad as he contemplates his new life and all that he has lost. But it is the emotion of depression which is causing him the greatest difficulty. Day and night, he is bombarded with thoughts of how much of a failure he is, how he is now different from colleagues who are happily ensconced in their relationships. How could he have messed up his own relationship so badly? He now believes that he is of less value than others. He can see why Olive would move on to someone more worthwhile. The kids continue to give some respite from these inner voices. They love their dad unconditionally, even if they are constantly asking when is he coming home, which breaks his heart.

Friends and colleagues encourage him to begin dating again, to put his separation behind him and move on. But he finds himself doing the opposite, withdrawing more, spending increasing periods at home on his own. He begins to drink excessively, to blot out the reality of his new, changed life. He eats junk food, ceases exercise and puts on stones in weight. The more this happens, the more emotionally depressed he becomes. There are times when he wonders if it is worth continuing. What is the point? He is going nowhere fast, a nobody, with the rest of his life an endless desert. At times his thoughts become darker, but he accepts that such a decision will destroy his kids for life and for their sake he pushes such ideas aside.

It is only a chance visit by an old friend, Vivian, who has heard of his difficulties, that helps Philip turn matters around. She is of a similar age and has experienced a separation herself. She, with the assistance of counselling, has learned to survive and now shares what she has learned with him. Her situation had been less complex as there were no children involved, but this did not make her separation any less painful.

She shares with Philip how writing down what had happened and pragmatically analysing it had been of great assistance to her. With Vivian's help, he applies our pragmatic blueprint, to great effect.

These were Philip's findings:

1. **How is this situation making me feel?**
    'This painful break-up has resulted in me becoming emotionally depressed.'

2. **What is it about this situation that is causing me to feel this way?**

'I am feeling down as I see myself as a failure as I have been unable to hold on to my relationship. I also believe that I am abnormal as I am now single and detached from so many of the relationships that formed a key part of my social world. I believe that I have failed my kids and let them down. I cannot see any future for myself and no longer see myself as a useful part of society. I am going to struggle to meet someone like Olive again and don't believe that I deserve to do so anyway, having let her go. Olive was right to leave, as I now understand that I am not worth much as a person to begin with.'

3. **What in my thinking is preventing me from dealing with this situation?**

'Because Olive has left me and I feel that I have failed in both my role as a husband and a father, I now believe that I am useless, abnormal, worthless and a failure. All of these judgements do seem harsh when I put them down on paper, but they truthfully reflect my opinions about myself at this moment in time.'

4. **What in my behaviour is preventing me from dealing with this situation?**

'In relation to my behaviour, it is pretty obvious that my lifestyle has gone to pot over the last few months and that eating junk food, piling on the pounds, drinking excessively and ceasing exercise are not making me feel any better about myself. Nor is pulling away from all of my friends and social contacts.'

5. **How can I short-circuit my thinking and behavioural blocks to deal more effectively with this situation?**

'In relation to my thinking, I need to reflect that there is little to be gained by constantly beating myself up as a person with terms like useless, worthless, a failure and so on. What do these terms mean when you examine them in greater detail? Vivian shared with me how these internal negative voices almost destroyed her, following her separation. It was only when, on the advice of her therapist, she began to accept herself unconditionally, that she reversed this process. Maybe it's time for me, too, to begin this process, to protect my own mental health and wellbeing. On her advice, I am going to challenge these negative self-ratings on paper and see if I can defeat them. I am still responsible, of course, for my actions and there is work to do there!

'In relation to my behaviour, I need to improve my diet, dump the booze, get out and exercise and put some structure and routine back into my life. I need to socialize more and break out of the negative cocoon that I have wrapped around myself.'

Let's discover what happens when Philip, following this pragmatic analysis, puts the above thinking and behavioural changes into action.

The easy bit relates to his lifestyle. He works with a personal trainer. Over a period of three months, his weight returns to normal and his fitness levels rise. He restricts alcohol to the weekends and only then with others. He reconnects with family and friends and is blown away by their expressions of love and support. Some share their own experiences following similar break-ups. He realizes that this is a commoner occurrence than he has previously believed. With Vivian's assistance, he socializes more. What begins for both as a simple friendship gradually blossoms into something deeper. Both, however, have been badly burned by their previous relationships, so agree to take matters slowly and see where it goes.

Philip is also becoming increasingly pragmatic in relation to his distorted thinking. Following months of challenging his negative self-ratings on paper, he begins to develop unconditional self-acceptance. He now understands that 'relationships fail, not people' and that it is often nobody's fault, just life! That it is normal, indeed increasingly common, for couples to split up and find themselves in new or blended families. It is also routine in such situations for children to spend periods of time with both their mum and dad. It is simply a feature of modern life.

He no longer sees himself as a failure or useless or worthless, but as a normal bloke who is doing his best vis-à-vis personal relationships and many other areas of his life. He now sees change itself as an integral part of life. Much of what happens in life is out of his control, so he ceases being so hard on himself when it, as is its wont, spirals out of control. He no longer responds by becoming emotionally depressed, but pragmatically deals with whatever issues underlie the change.

PART FIVE

HURT

9. Why Change Can Make You Feel Hurt

This section relates to those whose natural emotional response to periods of significant change is hurt. You may see yourself in this group, with hurt being your go-to emotion in such situations. Since life will throw up countless situations of change with the potential to trigger this emotion (such as demotion at work; losing your job; a friend, a family member or partner unexpectedly breaking off their relationship with you; or a row with a family member), you may find yourself visiting the world of hurt on a regular basis. You cannot dodge such life upheavals, so it's important to develop techniques to manage this emotion.

If you do not recognize this specific emotion as relevant to yourself, perhaps you may notice instead your behavioural responses at such times. For all behaviour has a purpose, and that is to satisfy some underlying emotion. The commonest behavioural response to hurt is to become hypersensitive or short-tempered with those whom you believe are partially or fully responsible for the situation you now find yourself in.

If you do find yourself residing in this space, you may wonder why you respond to difficult periods of change with hurt and behave in the way you do. The answer lies in the world of unfairness, a concept with which you may find yourself well acquainted! Let's explore this concept in greater detail.

The World of Unfairness

Underlying the emotion of hurt is the belief that you as a human being are being treated unfairly, either by others or by life. This irrational belief, as discussed earlier, often develops during your childhood, adolescence or young adult life. You begin to look at the world with a jaundiced eye, constantly seeking out situations where, in your eyes, other people or life are treating you unfairly. As with all unhelpful beliefs, if you only seek out proof from the environment that this is the case, then that is all that you will see, as you will block out all other evidence to the contrary.

You therefore begin to see everything that happens to you in life through the lens of unfairness, and periods of change are no different. This is an extremely personally damaging belief. You may notice, if you are observant, how you bring it into many areas of your life, especially into personal relationships. If your emotional response is hurt and your behaviour is to be hypersensitive, then trouble beckons on many fronts. This belief rapidly becomes an absolute demand when confronted with any negative change or occurrence in your life. This demand is that 'you should not be treated unfairly and that life should not treat you unfairly'.

But how realistic are these demands? Life, for example, is innately unfair and has always been so. Even the most cursory look at the world we live in confirms this painful reality. It is the poor and most deprived areas of the world, for example, that have suffered most from the devastating effects of climate change. The mindless destruction created by Covid-19 – as with so many other health issues, such as obesity, diabetes and heart disease – has also impacted more on the poorer sections of our society and world. Apart from the above, unfairness is manifestly prevalent throughout both the developed world (in the form of poverty, injustice and homelessness) and especially in the developing world.

It is glaringly obvious that each one of us will be exposed to unfairness throughout our lives. Much as one would prefer this not to be the case, the sad reality is that unfairness will be a regular companion on our journey. We therefore have to find new ways to deal with it. Many siblings, for example, have a different viewpoint as to whether they were reared equally or not by their parents. Many employees or managers may feel that their bosses are treating them unfairly in comparison with other colleagues. The list of potential real or imaginary slights is endless.

The Role of Your Behaviour

It is not only your belief and demands related to unfairness that can create difficulties for you, if you are exposed to some negative change in your life. It is also how you respond behaviourally to this emotion.

Human beings are like flowers. The latter blossom in the warm and gentle rays of the sun and shrivel when faced with cold, bleak winds. Human beings are similar. Each one of us responds best to openness, positive empathy and warmth. Likewise, we tend to respond negatively if met with suspicion, negative empathy, coldness or hypersensitivity.

It should come as little surprise, therefore, that your behavioural responses to hurt tend to deeply affect those with whom you come in contact. If you find yourself constantly suspicious of others, prickly, hypersensitive or sullen and broody about any comments or actions which you believe are unfair, then trouble beckons.

These behaviours may often trigger others in turn to view you in an equally negative manner.

You may then find yourself in a negative spiral. The more you demand that others and life should never treat you unfairly, the more your resulting negative behavioural responses will drive family, friends or colleagues further away from you. This in turn just strengthens your belief that 'they are all out to get me', triggering further hurt.

The negative responses of others to your unhealthy behaviours can also lead to them treating you differently, which usually finishes with you suffering the consequences of your own actions. You can learn new ways of thinking and behaving to ditch your hurt when some significant change in your life appears. Let's see how this would work in practice.

10. How to Manage Your 'Change' Hurt

The Pragmatic Approach to Managing Your Hurt

The pragmatic approach to managing hurt is to firstly question how realistic or achievable is your demand never to be treated unfairly by others or life. From our previous discussion, this is an unachievable goal. Life is unfair, so all of us will experience its lash from time to time, some more than others. People, too, have no intention of changing their behaviour in many cases, even if it is causing you hurt. Sometimes this behaviour may be intentional, but often it is not – simply people being unthinking or thoughtless in their actions. The pragmatist would accept this reality from the beginning. It would be preferable and indeed wonderful if either people or life decided never to treat us unfairly, but this is both unrealistic and unlikely to happen any time soon.

Pragmatism would also argue that carrying a hurt is like carrying a grudge against the person or against life, and that this grudge only harms ourselves. As previously explored, when discussing unconditional self-acceptance, human beings cannot be rated, only their actions. The smarter approach would therefore be to cease carrying a personal grudge against a person, for example, but focus instead on challenging their behaviour, a more constructive road to travel. Human beings dislike being challenged in relation to their actions or behaviours, so are more likely to change them if challenged.

However, the pragmatist would also accept that there will be times in life when people are not prepared to change their actions, even if confronted with them. Sometimes we have to either accept this reality or break off further communications with that person. We will see this understanding being played out in some of the cases which follow.

The pragmatist would also challenge whether negative behaviours, such as hypersensitivity or losing your cool with others, help you or alter the situation. It might be more useful to focus on the real cause of the problem, namely how another person's actions have impacted on your life and what practical steps you might take to alleviate this.

If you can see yourself in the above, it's time to change this narrative for good. The simplest way of achieving this goal is to apply our five-question pragmatic blueprint to such situations.

Family Dynamics

Let's apply this blueprint to one of the commonest examples of change leading to the emotion of hurt, namely the world of family dynamics. As Aoife in our first case (and Alan in our second) are about to discover, family dynamics can be complex, and a common cause of emotional distress.

Every family unit is unique, as are the members of that unit. Each member will have a different personality and viewpoint on life. While many families find a way to absorb all of these viewpoints and work as a unit to solve issues which arise, others can really struggle. It would be my experience over decades that family dynamics are a common source of hurt. Issues that may arise relate to sibling rivalry, money, wills, land, caring for parents and abuse, to name but a few. Sometimes families can split apart as a result of these issues and how they affect those involved. The risk of this happening is often greatest when some significant unexpected change enters the picture. Aoife's story, which involves a decision as to how best to care for a parent whose medical situation suddenly changes, is a prototype of the difficulties that often arise during such periods. Let's see how it unfolds.

Aoife's Story

Aoife's life is turned upside down when her mum, with whom she has resided for over a decade, suffers a massive stroke affecting her movement and speech, requiring significant long-term care. It becomes clear to both Aoife and her mum's medical and nursing teams that even with a care package, it will be impossible to care for her mum at home. She is completely unprepared for what follows.

Aoife, single and working as a dental assistant, has two sisters and a brother. To her surprise, they turn on her when she introduces the possibility of her mum having to go into long-term nursing care. Is it not the duty of Aoife, as the person closest to their mum and single (unlike her siblings who have young families), to give up her job as a dental assistant and provide long-term nursing care for their mother? There are some nasty comments about Aoife inheriting the house in her mum's will, which she finds especially hurtful.

Aoife has always believed that she has been treated unfairly by everyone and by life. She holds a particular grudge against life and the fact that she has never been fortunate enough to meet that special person. It is inevitable, therefore, that this new situation and how her siblings are reacting to it would restart this cycle of hurt once again. She begins to lash out verbally at her siblings. This provokes an even nastier response, consolidating her belief that she is being treated unfairly and worsening her hurt.

There will be many of you reading this who can relate to the above family situation, which sadly occurs on a regular basis, as many GPs can attest. Let's discover what happens when Aoife decides, on the advice of her close friend Tina, to apply a different approach to her difficulties by using our pragmatic blueprint.

Here are Aoife's conclusions:

1. **How is this situation making me feel?**
   'My emotion is hurt.'

2. **What is it about this situation that is causing me to feel this way?**
   'I am deeply unhappy that my siblings are assuming that I am trying to dodge looking after Mum. This seems really unfair. The reality is that much as I would like to do so, her care needs are too complex to be met outside a nursing home. They are also quite happy to see me left with the situation while washing their own hands of it, claiming that they all have families or are too far away to be of assistance. It is therefore left to me, which is unfair. They are also happy for me to give up my job and my life to look after Mum, while not prepared to do likewise. This is so unfair. Once again, life is dealing me a bad hand. Why me?'

3. **What in my thinking is preventing me from dealing with this situation?**

    'I am demanding, probably irrationally, that I should not be treated unfairly by my siblings or indeed by life itself.'

4. **What in my behaviour is preventing me from dealing with this situation?**

    'I know that since this happened I am lashing out at everyone around me, but especially my siblings. I have refused to answer their calls on a regular basis as I am so hurt by their comments. Work colleagues tell me that I have become sullen and broody, and short with them and patients.'

5. **How can I short-circuit my thinking and behavioural blocks to deal more effectively with this situation?**

    'I have had a good discussion with Tina about my thinking in relation to this whole issue. Am I being unrealistic, for example, in demanding that I should not be treated unfairly by others or life? Is this not an unreasonable and unachievable goal? Is it helping me in my life, or indeed with dealing with the situation, to hold a personal grudge against my siblings, since I have to admit to myself that I am? Would it not be better to take the heat out of the situation and cease making this out to be a personal attack on me?

    'Perhaps it might be more useful to explain to each of my siblings individually why their comments are causing me to feel hurt, and explore instead how to come together to solve Mum's sudden deterioration in health.

    'In relation to my behaviour, I need to learn the importance of withdrawing from any situation where I feel

I am going to lash out verbally, for at least five minutes. This might take the heat out of such situations. I need to make others, such as my siblings, aware of how their comments are affecting me. I also need to work with them to problem-solve the situation. If some of them are unprepared to assist here, then I must get on with the task of ensuring that Mum will be properly looked after for the remainder of her days.'

As a consequence of Aoife analysing her situation in this pragmatic manner, she is able to bring matters to a successful conclusion. She has some frank but respectful phone calls with each of her siblings, explaining how their comments had affected her deeply and also asking them to work with her to resolve the issues. She is surprised at the outcome, with each in turn admitting how they had been wracked by emotions of guilt, trying to deal with this emotion by dumping responsibility for the issue on Aoife. She also apologizes for her own behaviour, and for being abrupt and short with each of them.

This emotional catharsis leads to a family decision to seek out appropriate long-term nursing care for their mum, with everyone agreeing to assist in the organizational and financial decisions required to make this happen. Her mum finds herself in a lovely home, chosen with her children, where she is now receiving the best of care, with Aoife a regular visitor to keep her company.

In the process of dealing with this period of change in her life, Aoife, through the judicious use of the above blueprint, has also developed new patterns of thinking and behaviour which allow her to manage subsequent similar periods of change without resorting to the cycle of hurt.

Now let's meet Alan, Helen and Rita, who are also experiencing periods of transitional change in their lives and reacting with feelings of hurt. We will explore how the pragmatic blueprint detailed above assists them in analysing the cause of their distress and discovering new ways of managing it.

The Fraught World of Inheritances and Wills

As most family doctors will attest, there are few occasions more guaranteed to cause upset than the reading of a will following the death of a parent. This is especially so if the information contained in the will is perceived by some family members as unjust. It can be a major source of anger, hurt, disappointment and frustration on occasion to discover that you have been unexpectedly either completely written out of the will, or only left with a minor inheritance. Matters become especially fraught when substantial amounts of money or land are involved. I have seen families tear themselves apart at such times of change. Some of the most bitter conflicts that I have witnessed, in over thirty-five years as a family doctor, have taken place around the execution of wills, especially where farms or land are involved.

The death of the remaining parent is like the changing of the guard, the passing over from one generation to the next. Sometimes this is a smooth and fair process, where the parent in question treats each child in their will with respect and dignity, ensuring that none of them feel hurt or rejected. But often this turns out to be the polar opposite. A time when the knives instead come out. Where a parent decides to reward some children and bypass others, for reasons frequently too complex to enumerate. Sometimes it can relate to a personality clash between the child in question and their parent. On other occasions, it can be seen as a way of rewarding those children who in the parent's eyes looked after them best, even if this is often untrue. Or where the parent in question has particular favourites. The list of reasons is endless. The larger the family, the more money or land that is involved, the greater the risk that this changing of the guard, this reading of the will, may finish with some offspring being deeply disappointed and on occasion extremely hurt.

The reading of a will can sometimes unveil previously hidden family tensions, sibling jealousies or unspoken hurts as to how one was treated as a child or adult by deceased parents or other siblings. You now understand where you really stood, in the eyes of the writer of the will! Families are complex organisms, each with an individual life of their own. Matters involving wills and inheritances become increasingly complex if blended families are involved, following separations or divorces. This increases the risk of some losing out when the parent dies, while others may thrive.

The hurt and damage caused to individuals, families and generations to come can be devastating if the will in question is felt to be completely unjust, unfair, or a source of rejection for those left out or poorly treated. This damage can spread into the lives and relationships of those involved, with far-reaching consequences. Alan finds himself travelling down this road. Let's now see how he rescues himself from this downward spiral. There will be many reading this story who will see themselves in Alan and can relate to what happens to him. You may be one of those.

Alan's Story
Alan is one of three children. By the time he reaches adulthood, he already has a chip on his shoulder about being treated differently from his siblings. His father is a successful large dairy farmer, a man who doesn't do emotions and who is renowned for holding grudges, sometimes for life.

From the beginning he and Alan clash, disagreeing constantly about everything. Unlike his other two siblings, Alan loves the land and is determined to make farming his career. There is only one problem. Alan is the oldest sibling but his dad dotes on his younger brother, Seamus. He also has a soft spot for his daughter Kathy, but barely tolerates Alan. The more he tries to reach him, the more remote his dad seems to become. To Alan, this seems grossly unfair.

As time marches on, Seamus, to the great disappointment of his dad, decides to study civil engineering and from there goes on to manage some large civil projects. Kathy studies nursing and subsequently moves to the other end of the country to work. Alan, on the other hand, continues to work alongside his dad, even if the relationship is at best strained. He confides to his mum shortly before her sudden death from cancer that he has always felt like the ugly duckling, the odd one out in the house, especially in relation to how his dad treats him versus the others. His mother tries to reassure him that this is not the case. Alan, however, insists on holding on to his strong belief that he is being treated unfairly by his dad. He brings this belief into subsequent personal relationships, with inevitable consequences, as girl after girl leaves him, unable to cope with his hypersensitivity and suspicion. He finally meets Susan, who breaks through his defences, softening some of his behaviours. Then his father suddenly dies of a massive stroke and, as so often happens in life, this sudden change throws Alan's world into crisis.

It is revealed that, following the death of his wife, Alan's dad has changed his will. He leaves the farm to Alan's older brother, Seamus; the house to his sister Kathy; and some stocks and shares to Alan. This news comes like a bombshell into the lives of all three siblings. Seamus, who has never been interested in the farm, is now unsure as to whether he should give up his current job to run the farm, or consider leasing or selling the land. Kathy doesn't want the house as she is content with where she lives, but doesn't know what to do with it. Alan is simply shattered. All his hopes and dreams have died. He has put his heart and soul into looking after the farm, and now feels deeply hurt that all of his efforts have come to nought. He resents his two siblings for taking from him what he believes is rightly his. But it is the grudge he feels against his dad that begins to eat him alive.

He considers legal action and begins to lash out at everyone, especially Susan and his two siblings. He becomes bitter and impossible to live with. Seamus asks him to stay on running the farm, till he decides what to do with it. Alan, however, is finding it increasingly difficult to stay, as he now sees no future for himself. It is also a constant reminder to him of how unfairly he has been treated by both his father and by life. He considers just upping and leaving Ireland and emigrating to New Zealand. The only thing stopping him is Susan, who is a real home bird and unprepared to make such a move. Despite his behaviour, she continues to love him and wants to make their relationship permanent. Alan finds himself lost, filled with bitterness, yet uncertain where to turn next.

There will be many of you reading this story who can empathize with his situation. How many people have suffered the experience of being unfairly treated in terms of inheritances and wills? There are only two options open to you, however:

succumb to the hurt and bitterness, or discover another way to manage the issue. This is what happens to Alan. Let's see what happens when, with the assistance of Susan, he decides to apply on paper the five-question pragmatic blueprint to his current travails.

Here are Alan's answers:

1. **How is this situation making me feel?**

   'My father's will, and his leaving the farm and house to my other two siblings, has resulted in me becoming emotionally hurt.'

2. **What is it about this situation that is causing me to feel this way?**

   'I am feeling hurt as I believe that from the outset (and for reasons I fail to understand) my father always treated me differently from my other two siblings. No matter what I did, he never seemed to recognize my efforts. Even though I clearly loved the land and the whole process and lifestyle of farming, he leaves the farm to my older brother Seamus, who has no interest in it whatsoever. It is so unfair. He also leaves the family home to Kathy, even though he knew that I had often expressed an interest in it. He leaves me some stocks and shares, but these seem like bits of paper and not solid assets, like the land. I also feel hurt by life. This is a sickening blow. What did I do to deserve all of this?'

3. **What in my thinking is preventing me from dealing with this issue?**

   'I know that I am demanding, seemingly rationally, that I should not have been treated so unfairly by either my dad, or indeed by life.'

4. **What in my behaviour is preventing me from dealing with this situation?**

    'I know that if I am honest that my behaviour has been unhelpful. I am lashing out at Seamus and Kathy. It is not their fault that Dad made the decisions he did. And as for Susan, I just don't know why she has stayed with me. I have been impossible to live with, grumpy, broody, short and suspicious of everything and everyone.'

5. **How can I short-circuit my thinking and behaviour blocks to deal more effectively with this situation?**

    'In relation to my thinking, and following some deep conversations with Susan, I realize that it is time for a rethink. Is it realistic, for example, to demand that I should never be treated unfairly by anyone or by life? On reflection, this is irrational as life is innately unfair. Am I not just holding a personal grudge against Dad for all of those years when he seemed to favour the others, especially Seamus, over me? Am I just continuing and consolidating this grudge based on decisions made in his will? Am I also holding some personal grudges against my siblings? Are any of these grudges helping me in my life? Probably not! They are just making me feel miserable.

    'Would it be more useful to drop the personal grudge against Dad in particular? I always loved the crusty old b-----d, despite his behaviour, and often wondered why he turned out the way he did. Do I want to finish up like that myself? I am, of course, fully entitled to challenge his actions, especially in relation to the farm, as I still believe that these were unfair. But as Susan has gently suggested, none of us are perfect, and all of us, including myself, make mistakes, even if this one by Dad is a real clanger. It is up to me, however, to discover some way out of the mess he has created.

'Would it also not be sensible to drop any personal grudges against Seamus and Kathy, as I love them both, despite the current mess? Maybe it might be more useful to work with them to problem-solve the situation?

'In relation to my behaviour, it is definitely time to challenge my irritability, moodiness, sullenness and being simply horrible to be around. Nor is it helpful to take off to New Zealand, just to spite everyone. This is unfair to everyone else, especially Susan, and would just making the whole situation worse. It is time to sit down instead with my two siblings and see if we can come up with some solutions to the conundrum that Dad has left us with?'

Let's now discover what actually happens when Alan, following this pragmatic analysis and with the assistance of Susan, puts the above ideas into action.

Alan calls a family meeting, where he begins by apologizing for his behaviour. He promises to change it, a promise he has already made to Susan. He also explains to his siblings the hurt he has felt as a consequence of his dad's actions, not just in his will but throughout the years.

Kathy then reveals a critical piece of information, which her mum had shared with her privately before her death. She had become pregnant with Alan before they were officially married, with their dad having spent the first ten years of their married life completely ashamed what neighbours or family members would say if their secret was discovered. As her mum had explained to

Kathy, there was little forgiveness in those days for anyone who 'crossed the line' in such areas. This explained why her dad had always treated Alan differently. His father had remained ashamed about what had happened, as he was a deeply religious person. The mere presence of Alan was a constant reminder of their 'sin'. This is a complete eye-opener for Alan, who begins to view the whole situation through different eyes, as he now understands his dad's behaviour, even if he is not in agreement with it.

At the meeting Kathy and Seamus express their own frustration at their dad's decisions in the will, as neither feels comfortable with how Alan has been treated. They, too, are now burdened with the decisions as to what to do with the farm and house. The good news is that Alan has by then discovered that the 'bits of paper' his dad has left him are actually worth 'significantly' more than initially thought.

The three siblings thrash out a new road map out of their dilemma. Seamus agrees to make Alan a full partner in the farm, with the profits shared equally. Seamus also agrees to employ a manager to help Alan run the farm, paying for this out of his share of the profits. This allows him to continue with his civil-engineering projects, which he loves. Meanwhile, with the assistance of the bonds and shares left to him by his dad and a bank loan, Alan agrees to buy out the family home from Kathy, who is delighted with this outcome. All leave the meeting with the belief that each sibling is now getting what they wanted from the situation.

A year later, the whole mess has been ironed out. Alan is happily working the land, now sure of his future. He and Susan are now engaged and plan to move into the family home when the modernizations have been finished. There is only one final task remaining and it is one that Alan holds off doing till all is resolved.

Eventually he finds himself sitting by his parents' grave and having a silent conversation with his mum and dad. He tells them that he loves and misses them both. He forgives his dad, explaining that he now understands why he acted as he did. But he also notes that his dad's actions caused him significant hurt and pain and that he needs to state this. The tears flow and the load is finally lifted. He feels emotionally healed. One of the most challenging periods of change in his life is now over and he has learned much. Never again will he travel down the destructive road of hurt if faced with such a similar situation. He would instead manage such periods pragmatically!

Workplace Dynamics

Let's now visit with Helen, who finds herself embroiled in another common cause of change-related hurt, namely the world of workplace dynamics. The workplace, like so many other domains of our life, can be fraught with internal upheavals, often caused by changes in company policies, re-organizational disturbances or personality clashes, along with countless other potential flashpoints. This makes sense as the dynamics of human beings grouped together in any setting or guise can be complex and prone to such crises. Then there is the individual nature of each person working in such situations, whether at employee or management level. Each person reacts to negative changes differently. Some glide over such periods unscathed, while others are sucked in emotionally, sometimes to their detriment.

Hurt is a common destructive emotion, often triggered by workplace disturbances. It always comes back to the concept of unfairness. How many of you reading this can relate to specific incidents in your own workplace, where you believe that you were treated unfairly, triggering hurt? This could relate to a belief that you should have received a promotion over some other colleague, that a manager is specifically picking on you, that your work is under-appreciated, or that you are at the receiving end of a gender-inequality issue. There is an extensive list of potential flashpoints that can trigger this emotion in you.

Unfortunately, the damage emanating from this emotion in such situations can radiate outwards to affect not only work colleagues but also personal and social relationships outside this domain. It can lead to significant unhappiness, interpersonal relationship strife and even on occasion trigger bouts of clinical depression. As the workplace is simply one of a number of domains in our lives, the tentacles of hurt can unfortunately inflict significant damage on ourselves and others. This is why, as Helen discovers, it is essential to prevent hurt growing legs!

If you can relate to the above scenario and indeed this emotion, you will empathize with Helen's story. Let's now see how, by applying a more pragmatic approach, she manages to escape from the deadly clutches of hurt. Many have found these insights life-altering.

Helen's Story
Helen is a twenty-nine-year-old civil servant, who is knocked off her bicycle while travelling to work in the city and suffers a fractured pelvis. She is absent from work for four months and is just planning to return when she develops bronchopneumonia. She now finds herself back in hospital with extreme shortness of breath. She spends some days in the ICU but thankfully begins to respond to IV antibiotics. Helen had previously been in a relationship for two years, but this broke up shortly before her road traffic accident.

She had been badly hurt on discovering that he had been cheating on her.

With the assistance of her mum and some good friends, she eventually recovers sufficiently to return to work. She returns expecting a warm welcome from her colleagues. What she discovers, however, is a totally changed work dynamic, and not one for the better.

For starters, her section has been absorbed into a larger one, with her previous manager moved on to a different post. Helen now finds herself working alongside a group of new colleagues, some of whom are none too happy to see her return. They resented the extra workload placed on their shoulders when she was ill. Others treat her as if she has been diagnosed with leprosy, giving her a wide berth at all times. She tries to explain to them that she has recovered from her recent illness and is no longer infectious, but their behaviour persists. Even former colleagues are treating her differently, which she finds especially hurtful.

It is her new boss, however, who presents the greatest difficulty. Her previous manager was a warm, inclusive, empathetic woman, who got the best out of her team. Alas, her replacement turns out to be a tough, ambitious, narcissist male, with little time for any show of illness or 'weakness' amongst members of his team. Helen, unfortunately, in his mind fits into this picture, so from the beginning he treats her differently from other work colleagues.

Helen finds herself working in a small cubby hole, half the size of her previous workstation. The workplace ergonomics are poor, so her lower back suffers. Her boss refuses to trust her with assignments of note, insisting instead on passing over tasks which he considers of lesser import. He constantly drops comments that he is unsure if Helen is able to cope with the stress of more challenging projects. When she challenges him on this (as her initial response is extreme hurt), he dismisses her with a wave of his hand, suggesting that 'perhaps she should seek a transfer out of his section'.

To makes matters worse, former work colleagues refuse to support her, afraid of getting on the wrong side of their new boss, who is known to be vindictive. She finds their reactions extremely hurtful.

Helen has struggled with hurt since adolescence, and the break-up with her previous boyfriend has compounded this. It is inevitable that her new workplace dynamic would trigger this emotion. She becomes bitter, short-fused with colleagues, family and friends. She frequently retreats into sullen silences at work, making her work colleagues withdraw further. The cycle of hurt accelerates, and with it her inner pain and bitterness. The more she reacts to the boss's dominating, dismissive behaviour, the more reasons he can find to sideline her. His unstated aim is to hustle her out of his department.

Helen soon dreads coming into work and experiences increased anxiety and a drop in mood. Her family doctor suggests she take further leave on medical grounds, but she rejects this suggestion, believing that it will only aggravate the situation. She feels trapped and increasingly hopeless. On some dark days, she even considers other roads, but knows in her heart that this would destroy loved ones, her mum in particular, so desists.

Her behavioural responses to hurt are now beginning to intrude into her personal life. She has met through a friend a male policeman, Pete, a good-humoured, empathetic man to whom she is attracted. Her suspicion and hurt, however, are an obstacle to this relationship proceeding any further. Pete often finds himself at the receiving end of her sullen silences, unsure what he has done wrong.

She finally breaks down in front of her mum, a wise and sensible woman, who has experienced much in her life, including the loss of her husband at an early age. She notes how life can sometimes throw at us periods of distressing change and upheaval, and clearly this is one of those. They agree that anyone would struggle with the loss of a relationship due to an affair, a bad RTA, a visit to a hospital ICU with pneumonia and a total change of work dynamics including a boss from hell. Her mum, however, is a real pragmatist. While there is little they can do to change her relationship break-up, accident or viral infection, perhaps they could review her current work situation to see if Helen can find a way out of her difficulties.

Helen and her mum decide to apply the pragmatic blueprint to analyse her current dilemma. Here are Helen's conclusions:

1. **How is this situation making me feel?**
   'The change in my work dynamics, especially in relation to my boss and work colleagues, has resulted in extreme hurt.'

2. **What is it about this situation that is causing me to feel this way?**
   'I am feeling hurt as I believe that from the onset of my return to work, I have been treated unfairly. Some colleagues avoid me as I have recovered from a lung infection. Others resent me for being away for so long,

even though there was little I could have done to prevent this. My manager from the beginning resents my presence. In his mind I am weak, prone to illness and unable to cope with the stress of any routine project. My work ergonomic settings have been made especially uncomfortable to encourage me to seek a transfer or depart permanently on medical grounds. I am also hurt that none of my colleagues, due to fear, are prepared to back me.'

3. **What in my thinking is preventing me from dealing with this situation?**

'I know I am demanding that I should not be treated unfairly by my boss or work colleagues. I have to also admit that I am demanding that life too should not treat me unfairly.'

4. **What in my behaviour is preventing me from dealing with this situation?**

'My behaviour, too, leaves a lot to be desired. I am irritable, bad-tempered, short, even sullen with work colleagues. It has even extended, and I am ashamed to admit this, to my own family, including mum and my siblings. Even Pete, who is a lovely guy, has been getting it in the neck from me, often without justifiable reason.'

5. **How can I short-circuit my thinking and behavioural blocks to deal more effectively with this situation?**

'In relation to my thinking, and following a frank chat with Mum, is it realistic to demand that I should never be treated unfairly by anyone, including my boss or work colleagues or indeed by life itself? As Mum and I agree, life is sometimes bloody unfair, as both of us have discovered to our cost! We also agree that it can often throw arrows at us, in the form of sudden, unexpected changes, such as her losing my dad so early in their relationship. Who am I to think that I have a monopoly on unfairness? Is it not more sensible to wish it to be otherwise, but accept that that is not real life?

'I can now see that I am holding a grudge about so many things. I hold a grudge against life for taking my dad away so young, against my previous partner for his affair, against life for throwing an accident plus a serious virus at me. In relation to work, I am holding some serious grudges against my boss and work colleagues.

'Are any of these grudges helping me in my life? Probably not! Am I not, as my mum would say, simply carrying a heavy burden on my back which is set to cripple me for life? Maybe it is time to change this. I am beginning to recognize that I am holding a personal vendetta against my boss and work colleagues, instead of focusing on their negative behaviours. Perhaps if I cease doing this, I might feel better about myself for starters? This does not mean, as Mum has stressed, that I should not be prepared to challenge their behaviours or actions, some of them clearly wrong, verging on bullying. Maybe it is time to take on some of these behaviours!

'As for my own actions or behaviours, they too must change. It is not good enough to challenge other people's actions if I am not prepared to take on my own. I am going to do my best to reduce my irritability, sullen silences and an increasing tendency to lose it if someone crosses me. None of these are helpful. Maybe I need, as Mum suggests, to withdraw for short periods at such times, calm down and then attempt to deal with the situation.

'In relation to work, it is time to become more proactive. Maybe it's time to chat to personnel about what is going on in our section and seek out their advice. Perhaps I need to quietly but firmly challenge the actions and behaviours of both work colleagues and my boss, detailing why their actions are causing me hurt, and request they change them. If this is not working, then perhaps I should seek a transfer out of this section to a new one or even change to a different company.'

Let's now discover what happens when Helen decides, following this pragmatic analysis and with her mum's assistance, to put the above into action.

She begins by working hard for the following months on her behaviour. It sometimes requires her retreating for five-minute periods from potential flare-up situations. She requires regular trips to make a cup of coffee or to the bathroom! She challenges herself to stop being sullen and, bit by bit, becomes increasingly sunnier and more tolerant, a change which does not go unnoticed by those around her. Work colleagues warm towards her, as do friends and family. It does no harm to her current relationship with Pete either!

She also works hard on challenging her previous tendency to make everything personal and focus instead on what really matters, namely other people's behaviours or actions.

She begins to gently pull up work colleagues in relation to their actions or comments if she finds them hurtful, and discovers that a surprising number are unaware of the effect on her. Many apologize and promise to be more sensitive and empathetic.

Relationships between her and some of her colleagues dramatically improves.

The major change occurs following a specific incident where her boss treats her inappropriately and refuses to listen to her concerns. Helen finally does what she should have done from the beginning, namely to have a long chat with personnel. This turns out to be a game-changer in relation to her current situation. She pours out her concerns and grievances and receives a listening ear for the first time. She is unaware, but other colleagues have also privately lodged some concerns with personnel. HR are especially annoyed at her treatment following her return from both a trauma and life-threatening pneumonia, and promise that matters will be looked into.

Several weeks later, without any specific reason being given for the change, her boss is suddenly demoted sideways into a different section.

A new manager is appointed, who immediately takes Helen under her wing. Her work situation dramatically improves. Her new boss turns out to be empathetic and believes in a more inclusive approach, rather than the autocratic style of the previous incumbent. After six months, they are so impressed with Helen's work that they promote her to work on major projects. Work colleagues who in the past would have been jealous now come forward to congratulate her on her new post.

Helen is also discovering that her new pragmatic approach to managing change or indeed any negative situation in her life is bearing much fruit. She finds herself at last trusting Pete and that relationship is blossoming. She now accepts her mum's wise maxim that sometimes relationships work and sometimes they don't. It is not about fairness or unfairness or success or failure. It is simply life!

The World of Abuse

Now let's meet Rita, emotionally hurt as a consequence of encountering one of the most profound life-changing experiences of all, namely abuse. In her case she has experienced years of sexual abuse at the hands of her father. Of all of the experiences that a person can encounter, there are few more toxic or damaging to the mind, body, soul and spirit than abuse of any form. Abuse can take many forms. It can be physical in nature. It can be emotional. It can be sexual, felt by most experts to be the most destructive. In rare situations it may include all three forms of abuse. In Rita's case, it is primarily sexual.

Many developed countries have gone through shameful periods of institutionalized abuse of every type, where vulnerable children in care homes run by both the state and religious bodies were exposed to the vilest of physical, emotional and sexual abuse. Ireland has to hold its own head in shame at its past, as do the USA, UK, Australia and New Zealand, to name but a few. Despite the presence of such institutional abuse, most cases of sexual abuse frequently take place within the family home. Sexual abuse by male or female parents or siblings can be extremely destructive for the victims, who are often children. Equally destructive can be the form of abuse known as coercive control, perpetrated by male or female partners in relationships, with the victim frequently living in constant fear. More subtle but equally damaging abuse can relate to online trolls, sex-shaming and similar abusive behaviours. Another form of abuse relates to the dark world of people-trafficking, where victims are often horrendously sexually and physically abused.

It is not possible to explore such a large subject in this book. We will therefore deal in this section solely with sexual abuse occurring within the home. Sexual abuse changes the life of a person, sometimes dramatically. In my many years as a family doctor, I have seen it leave behind a trail of destruction in people's lives. It can be one of the most powerful predisposing factors leading to future bouts of clinical depression. Adult women, for example, who are victims of childhood abuse have been shown to be twice as likely to develop clinical depression. It is also a common predisposing factor in eating disorders, with adult victims having four times the risk of those who did not suffer childhood abuse. It is also directly linked to substance abuse and self-harm.

Sexual abuse of children can have a direct effect on the developing brain. At the time of the abuse, the stress of the event can cause the production of large amounts of our stress hormone glucocortisol together with other stress peptides in the brain. These high levels of stress hormones attack the hippocampus, which is the part of the brain critical for the formation and long-term storage of our everyday memories. It is one of only two parts of the brain that constantly produces new neurons throughout our lifespan.

Normally, when something happens to us, this organ allows us to remember the event and its consequences, whilst the amygdala (discussed in chapter one) remembers the emotional memory. In sexual abuse, the high glucocortisol levels created by the event damages the hippocampus, which is why so often the victim struggles to remember on occasion the precise details of what occurred. The emotional part of the brain in the form of the amygdala, however, remembers the anxiety, panic, hurt, shame and depression – emotions triggered by the event. In the case of repeated sexual abuse, the hippocampus on the right side of the brain in particular may not grow normally and can by adulthood be sometimes seen on scanning to be smaller than the left side.

This can be associated with severe lifelong bouts of clinical depression. All of this information is important, as we will discover when we hear Rita's story.

One of the most common emotions that victims of domestic childhood sexual abuse experience, apart from shame, is that of hurt. This can be extreme, profound and immensely damaging to the person and their ongoing relationships. In sexual abuse it is often found in association with depression and shame. For the purposes of our discussion in this chapter, we will focus on the emotion of hurt.

One would assume that in cases of sexual abuse the hurt is always aimed at the abuser, who has robbed the person of their childhood, their sense of self and often their future. Paradoxically, while this is sometimes present, the more common emotion towards the abuser is anger. The hurt is reserved for those who did not protect them from the abuser, or who claim that they were completely unaware what was going on. As we will see with Rita, she feels anger towards the perpetrator but is extremely hurt by the failure of others to protect her at such a vulnerable stage of her childhood.

In terms of change, it is obvious that sexual abuse itself is a life-changing transitional moment in the victim's life. But equally, trouble may emerge later, when the adult begins finally to investigate, challenge and deal with the consequences of their abuse. If it is discovered at this stage that someone was aware of or should have been aware of what was happening, and did nothing to prevent it, powerful emotions of hurt can be triggered. Unfortunately, the damage emanating from this emotion is rarely confined to the person who has experienced hurt from abuse, but spreads rapidly to include interpersonal relationships of all types, family, friends and intimate personal relationships.

Some of this damage is done through embracing a series of unhealthy, negative behaviours, which allows the hurt to grow legs. These, as we have seen, can include disordered eating patterns, misuse or abuse of alcohol or substances, becoming distrustful and hypersensitive in personal and other relationships or self-harm in the form of cutting or, on occasion, suicide attempts. Many of these behaviours are secondary to a strong belief that you have been unfairly treated by others and life, together with a form of self-loathing related to feelings of depression dealt with in previous chapters.

If you, like so many others, can relate to the above or have experienced any form of abuse, especially sexual abuse, and are really struggling with the emotion of hurt and its consequences, you may see yourself in Rita's story. If this is the case, you may find it beneficial to seek out some expert or professional assistance to deal with the fallout, and I would strongly encourage you to do so. Hopefully you may also find it useful to apply our pragmatic blueprint to your current situation. You are not obliged to live in the deadly shadow of your abuser or broken relationships. You are not doomed to self-destructive behaviours as a means of self-soothing your emotional distress. You can instead become free of the tentacles of both abuse and hurt. You can turn a destructive period of change into a potential period of growth. Let's see how Rita manages to do just that.

Rita's Story
Rita is a twenty-three-year-old college student who hits a wall on entering her final year, succumbing to a bout of significant clinical depression. Her friends are not surprised to see her crash as she has been on a path to self-destruction

for years. It was only a question of when, rather than if, she ran into difficulties. Rita has a complex former history.

She was initially a happy and carefree child, the youngest of three siblings, who seemed to be the apple of her parents' eyes. But as many family doctors are all too aware, none of us really know what goes on behind closed doors. Rita has always worshipped her father, especially as a small girl. As far as she was concerned, he was her hero and could do no wrong. Her father is a high-ranking policeman, regarded by the community as a fine, upstanding man.

The abuse begins when Rita turns eight and continues until she is almost eleven. At the time she is confused, not really understanding what her father is doing to her or why he does what he does, but she assumes that this happens to all children. Sometimes it really hurts physically and she breaks down crying. Her dad at such times tells her how much he loves her and showers her with gifts. Rita learns how to slip into an imaginary world when it is happening and this seems to help.

The words 'sexual abuse' are terms she comes to understand at a much later stage, but at the time she lacks the words or insight to explain what is going on. She tries to bring up the subject with her older siblings, but they just dismiss her as being childish. Her dad has banned her from mentioning it to her mum, explaining that it is their little secret. Then, for no obvious reason, around her eleventh birthday it suddenly ceases and her father withdraws from her, becoming an increasingly distant figure.

From then on, Rita is a changed child. She loses her carefree manner, becoming increasingly anxious and fearful. She blocks out the details and memories of everything that has happened but can't dampen down the emotional impact of her dad's abuse. In her teens she has a brief struggle with anorexia and also begins to cut herself regularly, to relieve her feelings of shame, disgust with her body and overwhelming panic attacks and anxiety. She begins to drink alcohol heavily in her mid-teens and even tries some weed to self-soothe. By sixteen she has gone through one significant bout of low mood, later diagnosed as depression, but does not share how she is feeling with anyone.

When Rita is seventeen, her father dies suddenly of a major heart attack. Rita finds herself conflicted about his passing. At one level, she grieves his loss, as he was her dad and she still loves him. At another level, she experiences a strange sense of relief but struggles to explain why this should be the case, as she is still successfully blocking out all memories of her abuse. She does notice that her older sister Anne seems to be reacting in a similar manner. Following his death, relations between herself and her mum and two siblings deteriorate and it is a relief to head off to college to begin her new course.

At college, however, things do not get any better. Rita scrapes through the first three years, barely passing her exams. She becomes increasingly sexually active, not really caring about who her partner is. She drinks heavily and experiments with every type of drug, but none of these substances block out her inner pain. She is now experiencing some flashbacks to what happened with her dad, but tries to suppress them. A close friend in whom she confides suggests counselling, but Rita can't bear the thought of sharing her inner thoughts with anyone else.

What triggers her current bout of major depression, however, is a chat with her older sister Anne on one of her visits home. Anne reveals that she, too, was sexually abused by their dad and is now receiving professional assistance to deal with it. She also reveals that their mum knew about his predatory activities all along but had chosen to look the other way. Anne has discovered this on confronting her mum on the advice of her therapist.

Rita then shares her experiences, a distressing conversation for both. Anne also notes that for some reason their middle sibling Eimear, according to a chat with her, has never been abused. This revelation makes Rita and Anne even more upset, although relieved that Eimear has been spared.

This conversation with Anne is a negative life-changing moment for Rita. She becomes consumed with a mixture of anger at her dad and extreme hurt towards her mum and to a lesser extent her older sister for not protecting her from their dad's actions.

Rita descends into a deep depression, requiring a prolonged stay in hospital following a serious suicide attempt, as she just wants to finally end the pain. With the assistance of the mental-health team and an excellent therapist, she begins to recover from this bout. She has to defer her final college year on medical grounds and is now on medication.

When Rita has sufficiently recovered, her therapist does some work with her on the trauma of her childhood abuse. She finds herself slowly improving as a result of this therapy, but is still battling with profound feelings of hurt, accompanied by concomitant feelings of depression and anxiety. Her hurt especially is all-consuming. She struggles to even look her mother in the eye, and avoids staying at home, choosing instead to stay with her sister Anne. She becomes increasingly bitter and short with family members and friends, but especially with her mum.

Rita now begins to see how much of her life has been altered and changed by her childhood abuse experiences and resents this completely. The abuse explains so much of her behaviour. She now understands why she has struggled with body image and mild anorexia in her teens, self-harmed, abused alcohol and substances and engaged in casual sex in her adolescent and college years.

With her therapist's assistance, Rita learns how to deal with her emotions of anxiety and depression, using the pragmatic blueprint discussed in earlier chapters, and she finds this approach extremely helpful. They then decide to apply this blueprint to her hurt.

These are Rita's conclusions:

1. **How is this situation making me feel?**
   'My emotional response to my childhood sexual abuse is anger and extreme hurt.'
2. **What is it about this situation that is causing me to feel this way?**
   'I am feeling anger towards my dad, who robbed me of my childhood and adolescence by sexually abusing me at such a vulnerable age. I also feel hurt towards him that he chose to abuse me and Anne, but did not pick on Eimear, which seems so unfair. I also believe that my mum treated me unfairly by choosing not to protect me, and turning a blind eye to what was going on. Was it not her job as a mother to protect her own children from

abuse by her husband? She let Anne and me down so badly. I also believe that Anne should have done more to protect me, but understand that she too had been abused by my dad, so was equally traumatized.'

3. **What in my thinking is preventing me from dealing with this situation?**

    'I know I am demanding that my dad should be punished for what he did, even if this is no longer possible. Equally I am demanding that my mum, sister and life should not have treated me so unfairly.'

4. **What in my behaviour is preventing me from dealing with this situation?**

    'I know that my behaviour over the last decade has not helped my case. By trying to deal with my pain and hurt through drinking, drugs, self-harming and casual sex, I am worsening my own situation. I have added to the damage done by my father and mother's behaviour. By refusing also to meet up with Mum and blocking her out of my life, I am not dealing with the issue which is causing me so much distress and hurt.'

5. **How can I short-circuit my thinking and behavioural blocks to deal more effectively with this situation?**

    'In relation to my thinking, I can now see that my demand that everyone, including my mum, sister and indeed life, should not treat me unfairly is an impossible one to achieve. Life, as Anne often says, is unfair. Both of us would have preferred if Dad had not abused us and that Mum had protected us, as this was her function as a mother. I also accept that I am holding some serious grudges here. I am holding a massive grudge against my dad for his abusive behaviour, but an even bigger one against my mum for not protecting me.

'But as Anne has suggested, perhaps I am just adding to my own burdens by holding a personal vendetta or grudge against them both. Would it not be better to forgive both of them as human beings, to drop this load and focus instead on challenging their behaviour or actions? This might mean a serious chat with Mum. Maybe this is long overdue! I long to also have such a conversation with Dad and to fill him in on just how damaging his actions have been to my life. Alas, he is gone. Perhaps as my therapist has suggested, I need to write down how I feel in a letter and bring it to his grave.

'In relation to my own behaviour, it is time to move on with my life. I need to cease misusing alcohol, food, drugs and casual sex as a coping mechanism to deal with my pain and focus instead on some positive actions.'

Let's now explore out what happens when Rita decides, following this pragmatic analysis and with her therapist's and Anne's assistance, to put the above into action.

She begins by working hard on her lifestyle. Out go alcohol, drugs and casual sex. In come exercise, a sensible eating plan and a decision to socialize in a healthier manner.

She has that meeting with her mum. There are some harsh words and a lot of tears shed, but at last Rita gains some insight into just what had been going on. It turns out that her dad had been horrendously abused physically and sexually by a predatory priest at boarding school, and that this had changed him into the abuser he became. Her mum admits that she was horrified on discovering that Anne was being abused and had indeed challenged her husband. He desisted from further abuse. She had kept a close eye on Eimear but began to relax when no abuse happened to her. This explained why she had escaped. But her father secretly re-started his abusive behaviour once again with Rita, managing to hide it from his wife for some time. It was only when her mum noticed Rita's demeanour changing that she once again challenged her husband, who admitted to his abuse. She gave him a final ultimatum and he never again bothered Rita.

When Rita questions why she had never come forward publicly to press charges against her husband, or to leave him, her mum breaks down. She admits that shame and the knowledge that her husband would lose his job and most likely go to jail had prevented her from doing the right thing. To this day she still regrets these decisions and begs Rita's forgiveness for her actions. 'I should have left him at the beginning,' she admits, 'but I felt sorry for him and stayed. I now know this was the wrong decision. Despite everything, I still love him, and I felt that he, too, had been the victim of terrible abuse. In some senses we were all victims, and still are, of that original abuse,' she adds sadly.

This conversation is a life-changing one for Rita, who embraces her mum, telling her that she forgives her. Together they cry, letting go of years of hurt and emotional distress, leading to an important moment of emotional healing for both. They vow that this cycle of abuse will now be broken once and for all. This leads to the beginning of a completely new relationship between the three siblings and their mum.

There was one other task for Rita to achieve. She writes a powerful, frank and challenging letter to her dad. In it, she details how his abuse almost destroyed her life. How she is now making him aware of the fact that his actions have taken away her childhood, leaving her with burdens of anger and hurt. She admits that she now has a clearer understanding as to why he became an abuser, but is still not prepared to forgive him for his actions, which were reprehensible. She does, however, still forgive him in the letter as a person and admits that she still loves him as her dad and hopes that he has found some happiness and peace, in whatever place he has gone to.

She brings the letter to his grave. With tears flowing down her face, she reads it out aloud to him. She then burns it, scattering the ashes over his grave. With this action, her hurt is gone, the burden is lifted and she is suddenly free for the first time since her abuse. It is over.

PART SIX

SHAME

11. Why Change Can Make You Ashamed

This section relates to those whose natural response to periods of negative change is to trigger the emotional response of shame. Maybe you, too, can relate to this emotion when some distressing change enters your life. There can be many potential causes for such change. It can relate to the arrival of a mental-health problem in your life, such as a bout of severe anxiety or clinical depression. It may be the loss of a job and the status that can go with this. It may be related to the arrival of cancer in your life, with you believing that others will look at or treat you differently.

It can also relate to making some major public gaffe or finding yourself at the butt end of social-media shaming, frequently completely unjustified. It may be that you finally accept that you are gay and feel ashamed as to what others may think of you. You may have been the victim of abuse which is now coming to the surface. You may find yourself suddenly in deep financial difficulty and ashamed that others will find out. The list is endless, as life can regularly, sometimes unexpectedly, throw up such occasions, with a potential to trigger shame. If you can relate to this, you may wonder why this is the case. The answer lies in the world of rating, a concept we discussed earlier, in chapter seven.

Let's briefly explore this further by examining the world of other-rating.

The World of Other-Rating

You may remember from our previous discussion on personal self-rating how most of us fall into the trap of merging who we are as a person with our behaviours or actions. How we all love to play the rating game, where we rate ourselves high up on the scale if things are going well and low down if not. How, as a result, we allow our internal critic to persuade us that we are a failure or useless or worthless, etc.

Shame follows a similar trajectory. The main difference with this emotion is that instead of just rating ourselves negatively if something changes for the worse in our lives, we allow others to do the judging for us, with the judgement usually extremely negative. In such cases, we are 'loaning out' our internal critic to other people to beat us up emotionally. Shame is often associated with some secret information about ourselves that we believe would attract negative judgements from others.

The pragmatic approach to the world of other-rating is to challenge whether human beings can be assessed or rated at all, either by ourselves or others. The answer is clearly no, so why continue with this destructive tendency? It would also accept that our actions and behaviours are definitely open to rating or assessment by others if it is felt appropriate.

Pragmatism would encourage you therefore to develop the art of unconditional self-acceptance. This is where you learn to love and accept yourself for the beautiful and unique human being that you are, but take responsibility for your actions or behaviour. In this scenario, you are no longer concerned about what others may think of you as a person, but accept that they are entitled to make assessments or judgements of your behaviour or actions. You are of course entitled to defend such actions if you believe such criticisms are invalid.

The Role of Your Behaviour

How you respond behaviourally when change makes you feel ashamed can also add to the problem. There are many behaviours that you may recognize in yourself, which are so easy to fall into. You may find yourself hiding from people or situations, as you are afraid they will discover your secret or judge you negatively. You may spend countless hours ruminating and catastrophizing about what will happen if any of the above does happen.

Some may struggle with sleep, diet or exercise if they are overcome with shame. Others can try to use alcohol to blot out their worries. Or they might head down darker roads and consider more serious ways of solving the problems that the period of change in question is presenting.

The pragmatic view of such behaviour is to ask whether any of these actions are assisting in challenging your tendency to allow others to rate you negatively, or in solving the issues in question You have to change such behaviours, even if this is difficult.

12. How to Manage Your 'Change' Shame

The Pragmatic Approach to Managing Your Shame

The positive news is that you can learn new ways of thinking and behaviour to manage shame, if this is your natural 'go-to' emotional response to change.

Let's explore how using our pragmatic blueprint can assist you to manage change so that you no longer feel ashamed. Let's see how this would work in practice by exploring a common example where change may trigger shame, namely inappropriate behaviour at work parties.

Work Parties

There is probably a good-humoured book yet to be written on the emotional mayhem that can occur as a consequence of routine office parties. This is in some ways inevitable. The mixture of office dynamics, letting the hair down and alcohol can sometimes turn out to be explosive, as Eve discovers to her cost. Such parties are frequently held to mark festive occasions such as birthdays, retirements, promotions and engagements, amongst others. But one festive occasion stands out as the greatest potential source of trouble, the annual Christmas party. Shame can commonly be triggered by this event, as Eve discovers to her cost.

Eve's Story

Eve unfortunately becomes extremely drunk and makes a few passes at some male work colleagues at her annual Christmas office party. To her horror, she finds some compromising pictures of herself from the party are put up on social media the following day. She becomes extremely distressed, ashamed of what she has done, her head filled with the negative judgements which will be heaped upon her by others, especially family members, friends and work colleagues. She constantly ruminates about what others are thinking about her. It takes her days to pluck up courage to return to work, citing gastroenteritis as an excuse. She spends days avoiding work colleagues and family members and constantly checking her social-media feeds for further comments. She finds it difficult to eat or sleep, as she is so distressed about it all.

Eve eventually confides in a close friend, who suggests that she apply our pragmatic blueprint to analyse her situation.

Here are Eve's answers:

1. **How is this situation making me feel?**
   'My emotion is shame.'
2. **What is it about this situation that is causing me to feel this way?**
   'I feel ashamed as I have messed up badly by getting drunk at the party and clearly made a few passes which I should not have. These are now out there on social media for all to see. What will people think of me when they see what I have done? They are definitely going to be extremely judgemental in their opinions of me. I believe that they are right to be so. I am also worried that

211

others in a wider sense through social media will now judge me as a drunk and a flirt.'

3. **What in my thinking is preventing me from dealing with this situation?**

'The main blocks are my absolute demand that other people must not discover my secret, namely that I got drunk and placed myself in some uncompromising situations, together with my belief that others will judge me negatively and I must accept their judgements as correct.'

4. **What in my behaviour is preventing me from dealing with this situation?**

'I initially avoided going to work, and when there I avoided work colleagues, constantly ruminating on what others must think of me. I am also scanning social media too much, expecting the worst, and am not eating or sleeping properly, as I am concerned that others will discover my secret.'

5. **How can I short-circuit my thinking and behavioural blocks to deal more effectively with this situation?**

'I have to accept that I am just a normal human being who has messed up. I won't be the first and certainly not the last. I have to stop being so hard on myself and yielding power to others to beat me up. Maybe it would be better to just accept that each one of us is a special, unique person who cannot be rated or judged to begin with, but that our actions are individually and collectively up for grabs. Clearly, I have messed up here in my actions. Perhaps it might be better to own up to these, apologize to the colleagues in question, and then move on with my life.

'It would also be healthier to cease checking social media, which is just a cesspool of rumours and intrigue to begin with. Do I really care what these nameless, faceless people think of me? Surely it is more important to accept responsibility for my actions and focus more on preventing any future recurrence!'

Eve then puts her conclusions into practice. She faces up to her inappropriate behaviour and apologizes to those concerned. They reassure her that it was only fun and nobody thinks the worse of her for what happened. As one colleague wryly comments, 'There are few of us who have not found ourselves at some stage in your shoes.' She ceases checking her social media and works hard on learning to be more at peace with herself. She also ceases to worry about what others think of her, but now accepts that she needs to be more careful of her actions at such times in the future. This has the added benefit of making her feel happier in herself and less ashamed about what happened.

Now let's meet Tim and Monica, who are also encountering significant transitional periods of change in their lives and reacting with feelings of shame. We will see how using the pragmatic blueprint detailed above assists them to analyse the causes of their distress and discover new ways to manage it.

The Stigma of Mental Illness

Firstly, let's meet Tim, who, along with countless others, is struggling with the shame of stigma following a recent bout of mental illness in the form of severe clinical depression. There will be countless readers who can relate to the emotion of shame when an episode or bout of mental illness or mental-health difficulties suddenly sweeps in, sometimes changing them and their lives for ever. This change can have a profound effect on both the person involved and those close to them, as many of those who have experienced such episodes can relate to.

There are many different types of mental illnesses which can lead to this emotion being triggered. It may be a severe bout of anxiety or major depression, an episode of bipolar disorder or psychosis, an eating disorder or a relapse of OCD. All of these have one thing in common. That the person experiencing any of these often believes strongly that other people will regard them as weaker or different or weird or somehow flawed for suffering from them. This will often be the case in their minds if news of their illness reaches friends, colleagues, or even on occasion other family members. In relation to bouts of clinical depression, this stigma may even involve spouses or partners, who simply do not want to know about your difficulties in these areas. Tim, as we shall see, sadly experiences this reaction.

Stigma in relation to mental illness goes back for thousands of years. Mental-health difficulties have always had a 'shame' tag associated with them, strengthened and deepened during the dark days of psychiatry. Nowadays, thanks to the bravery of many well-known sportsmen and women and celebrities, the stigma associated with mental illness is reducing. However, it is still unfortunately embedded within pockets in the wider community.

There is often, for example, an unstated assumption that if you have experienced a bout of one of the above mental-health conditions, you are somehow weak or abnormal in comparison with the rest of the community. That you cannot cope with stress. That you cannot be trusted in the same way as 'normal' people can. That you should be treated differently. This is the basis of much of the stigma accompanying conditions such as clinical depression.

We never use the term 'stigma' if discussing diabetes or heart disease, so we have a long way to go in relation to mental health.

This stigma often extends to the families of those with mental-health conditions, who may feel ashamed to admit that one of their members is going through a bout of such an illness. It is especially sad if the person involved is a spouse. It is hard to believe that you could be living with someone you love and yet still be ashamed to share such information with them, for fear of what they might think of you as a person.

At the heart of stigma lie two emotions: anxiety and shame. The anxiety in stigma is often triggered by the irrational belief that mental illness is somehow contagious, and that those close to the sufferer might somehow catch the 'illness'. The primary emotion underlying stigma, however, is shame, with those affected often preferring to hide their condition for fear that others will discover their secret and judge them as weak or abnormal. Some conditions such as clinical depression feed into this narrative, as the sufferer is already living in a harsh world of internal negative self-rating. Tim, as we shall see, is living in this world.

The damage emanating from shame due to stigma can have a deep impact on our social, domestic and working relationships. How many of us struggle to return to work following a bout of depression, as a result of shame? 'How will my work colleagues look at me, if they know that I have been off sick with a bout of this illness?' 'Will they not look at me as being weak?' This belief, alongside reduced cognition, is felt to be an important cause of prolonged absenteeism following bouts of depression.

But the experience of shame and stigma is not confined to depression alone, as many of you are aware, but covers all the other conditions already mentioned. Applying our pragmatic approach to the stigma and shame such conditions can trigger can assist you to cope with them. We are now going to examine how Tim manages to do just this. If you can relate to the above discussion, you may find yourself empathizing greatly with his story.

Tim's Story

Tim is a twenty-nine-year-old high-achieving sales executive with a large multinational company, living with his partner Andrea in an apartment in the city. They have been together for three years and are living the dream. Both are high earners, extremely ambitious and love to party. Then life, as it is wont to do, moves in and Tim's world suddenly begins to fall apart.

It begins with the sudden death of his mum, with whom he has an extremely close relationship. Andrea has a sudden miscarriage and grieves in her own individual manner, which is to sweep away her loss emotionally and carry on as if nothing has happened. Tim finds himself surprisingly affected by the loss of their child. Meanwhile he hits a speed bump at work, having lost a major client for reasons outside of his control. His boss is unhappy and makes it clear that Tim is now on his 'list'. He becomes extremely stressed as events all around him are suddenly changing for the worse.

Tim's mood, as a consequence of these changes, suddenly plummets and he becomes exhausted, apathetic, even struggling to remember or concentrate on anything at work. He loses interest in socializing, food, even sex, which causes difficulties in his relationship, and his sleep patterns disintegrate. He berates himself as being useless and stupid due to his cognitive difficulties. Andrea, assuming that he must have developed some serious physical illness, persuades him to attend their family doctor. Following some investigations, his GP diagnoses a bout of clinical depression, suggesting that he might begin a course of medication and attend a therapist once the medication has begun to take effect. She also notes, based on his history, that Tim has probably experienced a mild bout of the same illness while in college, but had dealt with it himself, using exercise as a therapy.

Tim really struggles with this diagnosis, but following a good chat with his doctor accepts that it is a bout of depression and agrees that it would be better to deal with it. His doctor also suggests that he takes some time off work, perhaps a month or so, to manage his condition. Tim agrees to put her plan into action.

Andrea, on his return from the doctor, is having none of it. She has little time for anyone with mental-health difficulties. She, like her dad, has always considered such conditions as indulgent weakness. As her dad would say, 'Just get off your backside, stop feeling sorry for yourself and get on with it.' This creates an immediate split between them. Tim finds himself trapped between his doctor, who he trusts, and his partner, who regards depression as a personal weakness.

He chooses to begin his medication despite Andrea's comments that they are simply Smarties or placebos, and does notice within a few weeks that his mood is improving. The medication creates further problems with intimacy, however, worsening his relationship with Andrea, who moves into a separate bedroom till Tim, in her words, 'pulls himself together'. He, as a result, becomes increasingly ashamed at having depression, which in turn triggers a further drop in mood.

He receives little sympathy at work either, with his boss implying by his tone that he, too, has little time for anyone with such issues and insisting that Tim should return to work as soon as possible. He also queries whether Tim is up to the task of taking on some upcoming major projects. He wonders whether these should be handed over instead to some of his colleagues, who seem to manage stress better.

Tim is now experiencing first-hand the reality of stigma. Maybe it would be better if he were to hide his condition from others such as family and friends. Maybe they, too, would judge him as he was now judging himself, as a weakling and weird. He vows to do just that. When Mick, a close friend, contacts him, querying why he is off work, he describes his absence as due to a physical condition and quickly changes the subject. So, too, with other family members seeking information on his current situation. Andrea, too, makes it quite clear that he is not to reveal to their friends or acquaintances that he has depression. 'What would they think?'

Relationships between them deteriorate further when Tim attends the CBT therapist recommended by their GP. The therapist helps him challenge his negative thinking, so endemic to depression. Tim finds working with her extremely helpful. Andrea however loses her cool, describing anyone who has to attend such a person as a 'loser'. Where has the man she moved in with gone? Once again he feels trapped, but on his doctor's advice continues to attend the therapist.

After eight weeks of treatment and therapy, Tim, his mood, energy, sleep and concentration a little better, is ready to return to work. But his feelings of shame as a result of the stigma he was experiencing have become increasingly stronger, threatening this decision.

How should he face his work colleagues and explain why he has been on sick leave? Should he just tell a lie? Should he simply tell them the truth and face their inevitable negative judgements for having suffered a mental-health issue? The more time passes, the more his shame increases and the more he delays his return to work. This leads to increasing criticism from Andrea, who just wants everything 'back to normal'. She wants the Tim she knows back, as she is missing him, but if not, she will have to consider moving out. This is the last straw for Tim. He even begins to have serious thoughts of self-harm to deal with his distress.

Thankfully, before his whole world completely implodes, he reveals all to his therapist. She suggests that they might apply the pragmatic blueprint to his current difficulties with shame.

These are Tim's conclusions:

1. **How is this situation making me feel?**
   'Because of my present bout of clinical depression and how I believe others are viewing it, I am feeling emotionally ashamed.'

2. **What is it about this situation that is causing me to feel this way?**
   'I am feeling ashamed as I believe that others, especially Andrea, consider that anyone suffering from a mental-health condition is a weak person, not to be trusted and different from normal people. I have come to realize that there is a real stigma associated with such conditions, unlike many physical illnesses. I am equally ashamed that my work colleagues might now discover

my secret as to why I have been away from work, and also judge me as being weak and untrustworthy.'

3. **What in my thinking is preventing me from dealing with this situation?**

    'I know that I am demanding that other people, especially work colleagues, friends, family members and social acquaintances, do not discover why I have been out on sick leave, for if they do, they will judge me accordingly, a judgement that I will have to accept.'

4. **What in my behaviour is preventing me from dealing with this situation?**

    'In terms of my behaviour, I know that I am hiding away from everyone, refusing to answer calls or social-media contacts from friends and family. I am finding excuses why I cannot return to work, though I am anxious to do so. I am also struggling to have a real conversation with Andrea, and to thrash out our future, which has been so disrupted by her views on my mental-health difficulties.'

5. **How can I short-circuit my thinking and behavioural blocks to deal more effectively with this situation?**

    'In relation to my thinking, I need, as my therapist has suggested, to challenge myself as to why I am bothered at all about what other people think of me as a person, irrespective of whether I have a mental-health condition or not. Am I not falling into the same trap which she and I have discussed earlier, of believing that human beings can be rated or judged in such a manner? I need to examine just how rational it is to blame myself, or allow others to do so, for an illness of any type. Would I be so upset if my work colleagues, for example, discovered that I have high blood pressure? Of course not. So what is different about depression? It is the illness which is abnormal, not me. I did not choose to get it, nor am I happy to have it, but someone with a migraine might feel the same. Perhaps the difficulties lie more with society and not with me!

'Maybe it is time to develop, as my therapist has suggested, unconditional self-acceptance, where I refuse to play the rating game or allow others to play it with me. Where I am happy to accept and love myself for just being me. If others struggle with this, it is their problem, not mine. I cannot be defined as a person by whatever condition life throws at me.

'In terms of my behaviour, maybe it is time to take a different approach. I need to face Andrea first. I am not sure why she is so against any type of emotional or mental distress, but I need to have this out with her. There is little point in continuing our relationship if we cannot overcome this obstacle, as there may be more such times in our lives. I am also determined now to reveal all to my family and close friends, who have a right to know why I have been out of contact.

'I need to lose my fear of returning to work and being upfront with my work colleagues. If they have a problem with my condition, then that is their issue. I also need to challenge my boss and if necessary have a chat with personnel, as I believe his current approach to my situation and his subsequent behaviour is inappropriate.'

Let's now explore what actually happens when Tim decides, following this pragmatic analysis and with his therapist's assistance, to put the above into action.

He begins by having an emotional conversation with Andrea. He expresses his concern that she is now regarding him as a lesser person for having suffered a bout of depression. She breaks down in tears, admitting how she has always struggled in this area. Her mum suffered from severe bouts of depression. There had always been an atmosphere of *omertà*, or silence, in the house in relation to such episodes. Her dad simply couldn't cope with her illness, considering it weakness, and he had passed on his negative views to hopefully the insertion on the line above fixes this orphan.

Andrea had also lost a close friend to suicide in her mid-teens and has never forgiven her friend for taking, to her mind, the 'easy way out' of her difficulties. She has vowed to never allow any mention of 'mental-health difficulties' to enter into her life. She has convinced herself that only weak, non-coping individuals succumb to such conditions.

She has never before shared these insights with Tim, who now understands why she has been behaving in the manner in which she has. This leads to a long discussion on just how unhealthy it is to deny the existence of mental illness and other mental-health challenges, and how damaging this denial is to their relationship.

Tim explains how much he has learned from his GP and therapist about his depression, the biggest insight being that it was an extremely physical and cognitive illness, affecting both the brain and the body. This insight has a major effect on Andrea's understanding, which she now accepts has been shaped by her upbringing. They end up having a long chat about the world of stigma and how insidious and pervasive it is. They vow to break down such barriers not only between themselves, but also with friends and colleagues.

Their conversation has one other major positive outcome, with Andrea now revealing how she is struggling to cope with grief following the death of their baby from a miscarriage, and her attempts to suppress this. She, on Tim's suggestion, agrees to attend a therapist herself, to work her way through her sadness and regret.

Tim, with Andrea's backing and that of his therapist, informs close family members and friends, even ringing some work colleagues before returning to work to share details of his illness with them. He is astonished to discover that several of them have suffered intermittent bouts of depression. One female colleague admits privately to him that she suffers from bipolar disorder, but has chosen to keep this information to herself as she is also concerned about stigma. All of them wish him the best and offer any support he requires. As he shares with Andrea, the whole process has been a really positive empathy experience, which lifts his mood further.

In relation to his boss, he decides to tackle him head on, requesting a meeting on his first day back at work. At this meeting, he lays out his concerns that he might be treated differently, seeking reassurance that this will not be the case. His boss takes this on board and within a month of returning to work it is as if he has never been away, with Tim once again involved in major projects.

Nine months later, his bout of depression completely cleared, Tim is off all medication and has finished attending his therapist and now in a new space where shame and stigma are a relic of the past. He and Andrea are now much closer. She has, with the assistance of her therapist, developed new techniques to manage her grief and is now ready to conceive again. Tim has become a mental-health ambassador at work, someone to whom other work colleagues can come if they are feeling emotionally distressed. He finds himself surprisingly busy in this role!

Both Tim and Andrea have come through a period of change which could have ended their relationship and ruined their lives.

Embracing change by applying our pragmatic blueprint has not only assisted them out of their current difficulties but also made both more resilient for the future.

When Cancer Arrives

Let's now meet Monica, whose life is dramatically changed when cancer in the form of a breast lump suddenly arrives in her life. Breast cancer is the nightmare diagnosis that every woman dreads. At least one in eight women will develop invasive breast cancer during their lifetime and around 3 per cent will die from this illness. The majority, or eight out of every ten women affected, will, like Monica, be fifty years of age or older.

It is not only breast cancer that can dramatically change the course of our lives. Many types of cancer can have a similar impact, whether it be ovarian, stomach, lung, bowel, prostate or pancreatic in origin. Depending on the stage at which they are discovered and the specific treatments required to manage them, the negative consequences of such a diagnosis can vary enormously from person to person. While many of us are aware of the obvious physical fallout from this diagnosis, few dwell on the significant psychological and emotional impact that it can have on our lives. Almost everyone will understandably become anxious. Many of us will get emotionally or even clinically depressed from both the condition and the treatments required, usually major surgery, chemotherapy or radiotherapy. There is another hidden emotion that often lurks in the background, namely shame.

It is unsurprising that you might struggle with anxiety related to a natural worry, that the cancer may kill you or, at the least, destroy the fabric of your life. Nor is it surprising that you might struggle with the emotion of depression. This can occur if, when diagnosed with cancer, you begin to see yourself as somehow different or weaker than those around you. Many of those who have battled cancer describe it as like being part of a 'special club', where only members can truly relate to this experience. Those outside the cancer club who have not themselves encountered the experience may sometimes struggle to relate to those going through it. We have already dealt with these emotions of anxiety and depression in earlier chapters.

But why might you feel shame if diagnosed with cancer? The answer lies partially with stigma, which we discussed in the last section. Although stigma in relation to cancer is not as pronounced as with mental illness, it is still there, lurking in the background.

If you are struggling with shame in relation to the diagnosis and treatment of a cancer, the chances are high that you are worried about others finding out about your illness and judging you as different or abnormal. Above all, you may be concerned that they will now look on you with pity, or that you might be perceived as weaker or somehow to be treated differently.

It would be impossible to explore each cancer or look at the individual nuances or changes that each one can introduce into your life. We are going to use breast cancer as a prototype of them all. Since the vast majority of those suffering from breast cancer are women, we will confine ourselves to discussing this group.

The modern approach to the management of breast cancer is to use a mixture of surgery, chemotherapy and radiotherapy, with each person being dealt with on a highly individual basis. This will usually involve the loss of part or the whole of a year for the woman involved, with significant physical and emotional consequences. Her life is often changed irrevocably.

The psychological impact of the physical changes, secondary to the treatment of breast cancer, can be especially damaging but frequently overlooked. The loss of part or the whole of a breast, even with the promise of an implant, can have a devastating impact on many women. They not only feel different about themselves, but are also ashamed as to how others (both male and female) will now view them. Chemotherapy can also be extremely problematic as it will often involve the loss of one's hair, or alopecia. This may completely change one's appearance, once again triggering shame as to how others might view you. Should I use a wig or not? Will this make me look even more odd? Others may be concerned that other physical changes, such as loss of weight, resulting from treatment may also make them look different, and this too can trigger shame.

There will be countless women who can empathize with the above, having experienced breast-cancer treatment. You may be one of them. You may be just embarking on the journey or have completed it. You may be experiencing a combination of anxiety about the future, depression as you feel different or odd, and shame as to how other women especially will now view you. If you are, I strongly counsel you to seek some professional advice in the form of a therapist who is experienced in the area, to assist you with your recovery.

It would also be my hope that applying our pragmatic blueprint may also be of some assistance in helping you manage this distressing period of major change in your life. While previous chapters can help you deal with your emotions of anxiety and depression, my hope is that this section will assist you to manage your emotion of shame. Let's now see how Monica manages to do just that and, in the process, transforms her life for the better.

Monica's Story
Monica has just turned fifty when her whole world changes and implodes. She has always been an outgoing, happy-go-

lucky woman, married to Francis, a plumber, for twenty-four years, and is the mother of two daughters, both of whom have followed her into nursing. She has always been in reasonably good health, despite struggling with her weight for the previous decade.

Monica experienced an early menopause, beginning at forty-four, and has been on hormone replacement therapy for the previous five years. She still has occasional flushes and night sweats but feels she had dodged a bullet in comparison to many of her friends. Francis and Monica are a sociable couple who love going out with friends and sharing a bottle of wine, good food and plenty of chat. She also does some nursing part-time in her local hospital as she enjoys the camaraderie of both patients and colleagues.

One evening when taking a shower, Monica notices a lump in her right breast. As a nurse, she is immediately aware that it doesn't feel normal and attends her family doctor. She refers her to the local clinic, where following a mammogram, breast examination and biopsy, a diagnosis of breast cancer is made. Monica is devastated, as is Francis. The specialist recommends surgery, followed by oncology for possible chemotherapy and radiotherapy. He is reassuring in that he believes that there is no evidence, on further scanning, of any metastatic spread of the cancer beyond the local nodes, and that her prognosis should be good.

Monica is concerned about the possibility of requiring a full mastectomy, but the specialist reassures her that he is hopeful that she might escape with a local resection of the lump. Alas, when the surgery is performed, the lump is more locally invasive than expected, and a full mastectomy, with significant resection of local glands, is required.

Monica is devastated, almost inconsolable, following her surgery, even when the surgeon promises to put in a prosthesis at a later stage. She feels immediately physically different or, as she admits to one of her daughters, 'less of a woman', following the surgery. She becomes emotionally depressed and a little withdrawn. But worse is to follow. Nothing could have prepared Monica for just how tough the following six months of chemotherapy were going to be. Between the nausea, weakness and vomiting, her life becomes a constant battle to stay afloat.

But it is the alopecia, or loss of her hair, which really distresses her emotionally. She becomes increasingly emotionally depressed, now regarding herself as being different and less of a woman. She also dreads what others, especially her husband, friends and family, will think of her. Her biggest concern is that they might pity her, something she simply couldn't cope with.

She has always been someone who took pride in her physical appearance. The loss of her hair is a massive blow to her sense of self. The suggestion is made that she could use a wig and this almost crushes her morale. Has her life been reduced to this? What a choice. Either spend six months with her head shaved or wear an uncomfortable wig. Matters get worse when her eyebrows disappear. How can she present herself in public? She begins to make excuses so as not to face friends and family, as she decides to keep her head shaved and can't face their judgement of her new appearance.

By the end of six months, Monica is really struggling. She now faces a period of radiotherapy, five days a week for six weeks. This produces another raft of side effects. These add further to her weakness and fatigue, and she develops uncomfortable pain and local swelling, and further alopecia from her right armpit. She even develops some swelling in her right arm. This makes her feel even more abnormal. Finally she is placed on a hormone therapy. To her dismay, this too comes with a risk of thinning or loss of hair.

She finishes the whole regimen, exhausted and a shadow of her former self. Even though Francis has been wonderful throughout the whole process, he is unable to lift her spirits. He is concerned that Monica genuinely believes there is a real stigma to having cancer and is ashamed about the physical changes which are an inevitable consequence of her treatment. No matter how much he reassures her that he loves the bones of her, Monica continues to struggle. Her family doctor finally convinces her to attend a therapist who specializes in assisting those recovering from breast cancer. This turns out to be a watershed moment in her journey of recovery.

The therapist empathizes with Monica's story, reassuring her that her experiences are really common, even if rarely discussed amongst the general public. Countless women find the whole process enormously stressful, frequently destroying their physical and emotional wellbeing. Only those who have survived such experiences can relate to the assault on one's mind, body and spirit. Monica finds herself breaking down into tears, experiencing an immediate lifting of a weight off her shoulders with this information, together with the warmth and empathy shown by her therapist.

It soon becomes clear that Monica is struggling with the three common emotional responses to breast cancer: anxiety, depression and shame. This is completely understandable, as her therapist explains. Almost everyone becomes anxious as to what the future will hold for them in relation to the risk of their cancer returning. Many become emotionally and sometimes clinically depressed due to the stress of the treatment and the belief that they are now different and of less value to others. They deal initially with these two emotions, then finally move on to managing her emotion of shame.

Monica and her therapist decide to use the pragmatic blueprint discussed above to analyse her current situation.

These are Monica's conclusions:

1. **How is this situation making me feel?**
    'Because of the physical changes which my surgery, chemotherapy and radiotherapy have introduced into my life, I feel emotionally ashamed.'

2. **What is it about this situation that is causing me to feel this way?**
    'I am feeling ashamed as I believe that others, especially Francis, family members and friends, now regard me as different. Maybe they will notice my missing right breast. Maybe they will see obvious changes such as my hair loss, even if this is thankfully slowly recovering, loss of eyebrows, facial changes, loss of weight with loose skin folds, the swelling in my right arm and especially that I bear little resemblance physically to the attractive woman that I used to be. They will now see me as different, someone to be pitied, to be whispered about behind my back, or to be somehow treated differently. How I am no longer attractive as a woman, only a shell of the person I was.'

3. **What in my thinking is preventing me from dealing with this situation?**

    'I know that I am demanding that other people do not discover that I have had breast-cancer surgery or further treatments. I am demanding especially that if they do find out, they will not judge me as weird or ugly, or treat me differently as a result of my treatment for cancer, or worst of all pity me, as I would have to accept that their judgement in such circumstances is accurate.'

4. **What in my behaviour is preventing me from dealing with this situation?**

    'In terms of my behaviour, I know that I have been hiding away from meeting up with some members of my family, close friends and especially work colleagues. I know I have shut down all of my social-media interactions, which has isolated me further. I am spending too much time in front of the mirror, only seeking out my physical imperfections and trying to hide them in any way I can. This has led to me living increasingly like a hermit. I am also looking for any reason not to return to work, in case work colleagues, too, will begin to judge me negatively.'

5. **How can I short-circuit my thinking and behavioural blocks to deal more effectively with this situation?**

    'In relation to my thinking, maybe, as my therapist has suggested, it is time for me to begin exploring why I am so obsessed with what other people think of me. Am I not merging my assessment of myself physically with who I am as a person and therefore basing my personal happiness on their judgements? Maybe it is time, as my therapist has also suggested, to develop unconditional self-acceptance, where I refuse to play what she calls the rating game or allow others to play it with me. Where I am happy to accept and love myself for just being me. If others struggle with this, it is their problem, not mine.

'I also have to be realistic and pragmatic about everything that has happened to me since my diagnosis. I did not give myself my breast cancer and have to accept that the surgery, chemotherapy and radiotherapy were essential to save my life and to prevent a recurrence of the tumour. These treatments do have significant effects on physical and mental health, as I have discovered, but was there any other choice?

'I also have to be sensible and realize that the "real me" underneath these physical alterations has not changed, as Francis and my therapist have repeatedly reassured me. Is my beauty only to do with my physical appearance, or is it more to do with who I am as a person?

'If I accept that the above is true, is it not time to change my perspective on what has happened, and focus on the positive aspects? I am alive, weaker than when this regimen began, but now able to look forward to the future with Francis and the children. My hair will recover, if not as strong as before. The specialist has promised that later they will do some cosmetic surgery in relation to my breast and deal with the excessive skin folds.

'Based on this, is it not time to ditch my concerns as to what others think of me physically or indeed as a person? They are entitled to their opinions, but I am not obliged to accept them. If I truly accept myself as being special and unique, then all the rest is irrelevant.

'In relation to my behaviour, it is pretty clear what needs to be done. I am going to share my experiences with family, friends and work colleagues, and that includes discussing the effects of my treatment with them. I am going to return to work as soon as possible. I am going to try to live my life to the full now, and stop hiding myself away from others.'

Let's see what happens when Monica decides, following this pragmatic analysis and with her therapist's and Francis's assistance, to put the above into action.

She begins with her behaviour, which has been contributing so much to her difficulties. She makes contact with all those within her family and wider social circle and shares her experiences with them. She is greatly heartened when other women come forward to share their experiences with breast cancer. All of them comment on how much they have struggled, even up to this day, with emotions of anxiety, depression and especially shame. Some had never revealed their story and found it to be of great assistance to share it with Monica. As one, they all admit how the treatment has damaged their sense of themselves physically and emotionally as women, and to the multiple other ways it has changed their lives. This encourages Monica to open a blog where she shares her personal experiences and those of others. To her surprise, this produces a phenomenal response, as thousands of women contact her to share their experiences, many commenting on how ashamed they had been of their physical appearance, both during and following treatment. As she notes to Francis, sharing her own story through her blog has opened up a hidden wound in the community. Clearly, she is not alone!

A year later, Monica is in a new space. She has become increasingly acceptant of herself, warts and all, and has discovered that this period has also made her more empathetic to the suffering of others. She has had some cosmetic surgery and this, combined with a new fitness and dietary regimen, sees her glowing with health. Her relationship with Francis if anything has deepened, and they could not be any closer physically or emotionally. She has returned to work, heartened by the wonderful support she receives from her colleagues. She still runs her blog and has now expanded this into weekly podcasts, where other women share their stories. As she notes to her therapist, it is high time that girl power took over and women learn to assist each other through this most difficult of times.

PART SEVEN

SADNESS AND REGRET

13. Why Change Can Trigger Sadness and Regret

It is appropriate that the last part of our journey into embracing change will end with two of the most common and most powerful human emotions of all, namely sadness and regret. Although healthy negative emotions, as discussed in chapter one, these are emotions which profoundly affect each one of us on a regular basis throughout our lives. As the years roll on, sadness and regret become more poignant and meaningful as the great changes of life begin to take effect, in the form of ageing, loss and death. They are also common emotional reactions to periods of significant change throughout the whole lifespan. Almost every reader can identify such periods and the emotions in question.

The Role of Loss

Sadness is related to loss in all its forms. Some of the most painful periods of change during our lifespans relate to loss, so it is unsurprising that sadness is embedded in the human psyche. We shall be meeting Sandra, Damien and Sheila later, who are experiencing such periods.

*

Loss can present itself in many ways. The most profound relates to the death of someone close to us, but it can apply to plenty of common situations, many of which each one of us is familiar with. It can relate to the loss of a relationship either personal or familial, or the loss of a beloved pet. It may be a sense of loss for what might have been, associated with a diagnosis of a terminal cancer. Or the loss of a job from retirement, ill health or redundancy. It can relate to the empty-nest syndrome, especially if children travel far afield, or a loss of innocence from abuse. On other occasions, it may be a loss of physical health preventing us from taking part in sports or other leisure activities. In severe cases it can relate to a loss of partial or total function from paralysis or a stroke. It can also relate to the increasing loss of family members and close friends due to ageing, as Sheila discovers in her story. The list is endless.

At the heart of the healthy negative emotion of sadness lies the rational healthy belief or understanding that whoever or whatever we have lost is now gone, in some cases – as in the case of the death of a loved one – for ever. This loss can be associated with significant feelings of emotional pain and sadness. Loss is also often associated with a significant change in the lives of those left behind. If your whole life has been bound up with the person who has died, as is often the case with long-term couples, you may feel their loss deeply. Not only is the person you love now no longer with you, but you are also facing a life without them. This can often have dramatic effects on your social, domestic and personal life.

In the case of a personal relationship break-up, there is also the loss of both the person and the whole social framework you had built around them. This can induce great sadness. You are mourning the loss of what might have been as much as the person themselves. So, too, with a beloved pet. In the case of a terminal illness, there is also the loss of what might have been. Each of these situations involves significant change in the lives of those affected.

Sadness, in all these situations, relates therefore to the twin changes involved in loss. The first relates to the actual loss of the person, pet or life potential. The second relates to the loss of what might have been if the above had not occurred.

Sadness can be a deeply felt negative emotion, even if it is perceived as being healthy. It is completely natural for us as human beings to feel like this, if we experience an important loss in our lives.

The Role of Our Decisions

Regret is related to our analysis of some decisions or actions that we carried out at some stage in our life, the consequences of which turned out to be more negative than we expected. Life is full of those kind of decisions at every turn.

Regret is related to a realization as to what might have been if we had charted a different course at some stage in our lives. Or made some different choices or decisions. How many of us can instantly relate to such periods, where we would have preferred in hindsight to have chosen a different path or decision? I am sure you, too, can relate to such periods. Regret is less about blaming ourselves for what happened, as happens in guilt; more about wishing that things had turned out differently. It is more about a healthy demand that you wish you had taken a different course, now that you know how the decision worked out.

There are numerous occasions in life that can trigger regret. It may be the break-up of a key personal relationship for what turns out to be poorly thought-out reasons. It may be rows with parents or children or siblings, with this emotion sometimes aggravated if one or the other dies unexpectedly. It may be a career choice, where one wishes one had travelled down a different route. It may be a regret about not living life to the full and now, when older, being unable to achieve your dreams. Once again, you may see yourself in this list and frequently pine about such decisions.

Regret, like sadness, although a healthy emotion, can still be painful. How many of us feel wistful as to how decisions we made turned out? It is related to change, in that the decisions you made usually involved making some significant change in your life at that time. You are now regretting that change and wishing that the consequences of it were different.

I have chosen to put both emotions together as it has been my lifelong experience that sadness and regret often go hand in hand, and we will see this play out in the stories which unfold.

The Role of Your Behaviour

Sadness and regret can both be associated with healthy and, on occasion, with unhealthy behaviours. Let's explore some of these in more detail.

Our natural healthy human response to sadness is to shed tears, to cry. For some of us, this comes easier than for others and it is important that you must go with whatever feels natural for you. It is also natural and healthy to ruminate about your loss, to pine for the person or for what is gone, or for the future you might have had.

It is unhealthy, however, when you block out the loss, suppress your grief, completely isolate yourself from others, or try to block your sadness by diverting it to anger or guilt. Our natural healthy response to regret is to reflect regularly on the consequences of the decision in question, or perhaps on occasion to try to mitigate its effects on others in some situations. It is unhealthy, however, when you spend excessive periods of time ruminating constantly on the decision or action in question, trying to visualize how you could have done things differently. Or ruminating on the negative consequences it led to.

14. How to Manage Your 'Change' Sadness and Regret

The Pragmatic Approach to Sadness and Regret

The pragmatic approach to sadness is that it is completely human to feel this emotion when confronted with periods of loss during your life, irrespective of the cause. Sometimes it is useful to describe life as a series of losses, as that is an accurate reflection of what happens to each one of us. It is natural to mourn the loss of what was previously there, or what might have been.

Pragmatism would refuse to put a time limit on how long this period of sadness may continue for, as it is so variable from person to person and dependent on the depth of the loss sustained. It is therefore healthy, if extremely painful, to feel sadness at such times and better to accept that this is simply your emotional response to what has been taken from your life. This is especially the case in situations such as the death of someone close to you or the ending of a relationship. Pragmatism would also challenge you to see if your behavioural responses are assisting you in managing the situation or worsening it.

The pragmatic approach to regret is to accept that there will be many times in life when you will make choices or decisions that just don't work out. None of us can see into the future as to how such decisions will turn out. Let yourself off the hook, accept that what is done is done and move on with your life, sometimes much the wiser!

Let's now meet Sandra, who is feeling both sadness and regret following the decision of her youngest daughter to emigrate with her boyfriend to Australia. She is experiencing another of those major transitional change periods of life.

The Empty-nest Syndrome

As parents involved in the rearing of our children, the years seem to pass so quickly. Our task is to prepare them to become young adults, ready to take on the world. Sooner than expected, that time arrives when our children must go forth into the world to begin their adult lives, like fledglings leaving the nest. When the final child departs, it can initiate a period of intense change for parents as they find themselves in a house suddenly empty of noise and laughter. This period of change can lead on occasion to significant emotional distress. This has led to the term 'empty-nest syndrome', which relates to the emotional impact, and sense of loss and grief, experienced by some parents as their children gradually move out.

It is important to point out that many couples look forward to this time. To having more time to get to know each other again as a couple, and being free to travel. For others, especially for some mums who have poured much of their lives, time, effort and selves into the rearing of their children, this can be a difficult period of change, however. This is especially the case if it is the last child leaving. Or if the children departing are widely distributed world-wide, with some perhaps even finding themselves on the other side of the globe in faraway places such as Australia or New Zealand.

Emotional reactions can differ but, in many cases, there is often a mixture of sadness and regret as a result of this transitional period of change. This is what happens to Sandra.

Sandra's Story

Sandra is fifty-three, married to an electrician, John, and mother to two girls, Susan and Catherine. They live in a busy provincial town. Sandra works part-time in a local super-market. Her whole world has revolved around her two children, whom she idolizes, with those feelings strongly recip-rocated. Susan and Catherine both work hard and advance to tertiary education. Whilst at college, both return home every second weekend, so Sandra, although she misses them greatly, is still able to see them regularly.

But then life, as is its wont, changes the narrative. Susan announces that she is moving to California for a year or two, together with her American boyfriend, Zac. Sandra's spir-its drop as she contemplates the distance between California and where they currently live. But worse is to come. Cath-erine then announces that she is taking a year out to travel to Australia with her boyfriend, Ian, who has some family members living there. Sandra's heart is broken at the thought of both of her daughters being so far away. Both reassure her that modern communications will allow them to stay constantly in touch. Susan even suggests that John and Sandra might take trips out to see them at her expense.

Nothing, however, prepares Sandra for the emotional devastation that follows on from their departures, especially when Catherine, the youngest, leaves home. The tears flow copiously at the airport and continue unabated for the sub-sequent weeks and months. Sandra finds herself pining for their return. She struggles most on entering their bedrooms, suddenly empty of their presence. She misses their voices and their laughter. John does his best to reassure her that it will only be for a while. But Sandra in her heart senses that they will be gone for a long time, if not for ever, as both girls seem extremely happy with their new jobs and way of life. There are increasing hints about staying for longer periods in both situations.

Sandra finds herself feeling constantly sad, with John wondering if she is becoming depressed. She just can't see a future life for herself in their absence. She has heard some friends talking about the empty-nest syndrome and how distressing it has been for them. While other friends have spoken of such periods with glee, looking forward to spending more time with their spouses and on personal hobbies, this is not the case for Sandra. She has put her whole life into rearing her two children and with their departure goes her future.

She regularly admits to John that her greatest fear is that they will decide to settle permanently in the USA and Australia and that she will never get to see her grandchildren, if there are any, grow and develop. She regrets that she has not prepared better for this period by developing other hobbies and interests. Now she finds herself with too much free time to ruminate and feel sad at the loss of her children. How can she ever come to terms with this major change in her life? All she can see in front of her is a life of sadness, loss and regret. She finds herself withdrawing socially, comfort eating and piling on extra weight, making her feel even more miserable.

Finally, on John's advice, she attends a female therapist recommended by one of his friends. She pours out her distress at losing her children to emigration and her inability to adapt to her new situation. How she is struggling to get through each day. How she can't cope with the silence and the absence of that longstanding camaraderie which exists between herself and her two daughters. How the Skype and Zoom calls are not sufficient, often making her feel more alone and sad. How she can't see any future for herself. How it is causing relationship difficulties with John, who has a more pragmatic view of their departure. In his eyes, the girls have to move on with their lives and live wherever and in whatever manner they see fit.

Her therapist empathizes, explaining that Sandra is experiencing a common phenomenon called the 'empty-nest syndrome'. How this often affects women in particular as they frequently invest more of their emotional energies into rearing their children than men. She suggests using our five-question pragmatic blueprint to analyse her situation.

These are Sandra's answers:

1. **How is this situation making me feel?**
   'My emotions are sadness and regret.'
2. **What is it about this situation that is making me feel this way?**
   'I feel sadness because of the loss of my two daughters from my everyday life. This sense of loss has been heightened by the fact that they are living so far away, Susan in California and Catherine in Australia. Both are increasingly settled in their new environments and likely to remain there indefinitely. I am sad at the possibility that I will lose the opportunity of seeing my future

grandchildren grow and develop, if the girls decide to stay. I feel regret that having spent so much time rearing them, I did not prepare for this empty-nest phase and now feel completely lost.'

3. **What in my thinking is preventing me from dealing with this situation?**

    'The main block to dealing with my sadness is my inability to come to terms with my loss and accept the reality that my children have to progress in their lives in whatever form this takes, even moving to a different country. In relation to my regret, I would also have preferred to have prepared better for this scenario, but was blissfully unaware that this situation would evolve in the manner in which it did.'

4. **What in my behaviour is preventing me from dealing with this situation?**

    'I am spending too much time ruminating upon my situation. I am also isolating myself too much from friends and family and making no effort to adapt to my new situation. I am also comfort eating to cope with my pain and this is making me increasingly overweight, adding to my difficulties.'

5. **How can I short-circuit my thinking and behavioural blocks to deal more effectively with this situation?**

    'I have to accept that, much as I would like to have my children living close to me, they must each travel their own journey in life, wherever this takes them. I need to recognize that it is OK to be sad as this is a significant loss occurring at a real transitional phase of my life. I have to carry that natural sadness with me, but also begin to pick up the pieces of my life again. My life without the two girls will be different, but I have to adapt to this new situation.

'It might help to try to adapt the approach that this change opens up some new possibilities for myself and John, at both a personal and relationship level. I have to accept that the two girls are not gone permanently from us, but rather are just at a distance. They have also promised to come back to see us on a regular basis.

'Maybe it is time for a new beginning, to take re-sponsibility for my own life. I need to begin a dietary and fitness regime. I also need to look into taking up some new activities and hobbies. Maybe it is also time for John and I to take those promised breaks around Ireland. Maybe it is even time to consider taking a trip to both California and Australia to see them. What an exciting prospect!'

Let's now discover what happens when Sandra decides, follow-ing this pragmatic analysis and with John's assistance, to put the above blueprint into action.

Over the following six months she tackles her lifestyle, losing a significant amount of weight and becoming fitter and healthier. She decides to join the Tidy Towns committee and involve her-self in some local charities, especially Meals on Wheels. She and John begin to plan several trips to local and national beauty spots which they have often discussed visiting. They also join the local music society and film club and even take up Irish Set dancing. Catherine and Susan begin to joke with Sandra online that she is now rarely around to take their calls as she is so busy.

They also begin to save for the trip of a lifetime, taking in Cal-ifornia and Australia as part of a world-wide tour. Soon, Sandra notes that her sadness is gradually easing. She still misses her girls and looks forward to seeing them on their occasional trips home, but has now adapted to her new life, which she loves. Who knows, as she comments to John, what the future will bring? Whether the girls will eventually come home or not? Whatever the final outcome, they will adapt and cope with whatever life throws at them!

Ageing

Now let's meet Sheila, who is facing one of the most challenging phases of life, another period of constant change and loss, namely the world of ageing. Even our understanding of the ageing process itself is in a state of constant flux and change.

With improvements in health, science and technology, we are all living longer than our predecessors. As recently as the nineteenth century, the average life expectancy was low, between thirty and forty years of age. Nowadays life expectancy in developed countries such as the UK has climbed to over eighty, and is even greater in countries like Japan. By the time our children have reached this phase of life, average life expectancy will have climbed to the hundred mark. We are also living in a Western world culture where many populations are ageing, with increasing numbers of us reaching the age of sixty-five, and global worldwide numbers projected to triple to one and a half billion.

There is a tendency amongst public and media alike, when discussing the subject of ageing, to assume that it only applies to those over seventy-five. The reality of course is that ageing is a gradual process, beginning from fifty onwards; some would even say a decade earlier. The Covid-19 pandemic led to some heated discussions as to who we define as aged and more especially how they should be defined.

There is also a clear difference as to how ageing affects each individual person. Some of us will age at a faster rate than others, due to a mixture of genetic, lifestyle and environmental reasons. Some of us may, for example, be fit and healthy eighty-year-olds, fleet of foot, active cognitively and socially interactive. Others may be less so, struggling with cardiac, cerebrovascular, respiratory or orthopaedic issues, encountering difficulties with hearing or eyesight, or increasingly cognitively impaired.

This has led to the concept of your biological versus your chronological age.

What this means in practice is that I might be seventy years of age chronologically, but due to a mixture of genes and lifestyle have the functioning body of a sixty-year-old. This is why there is an increasing emphasis on all of us developing healthier lifestyles. Simple lifestyle changes, such as exercise, sensible dietary and alcohol regimens, focusing on our sleep patterns, keeping ourselves cognitively active and improving social interactions with others, for example, seem to slow down the negative effects of ageing on our bodies, brains and minds. This is an extremely positive message to get out there. You can greatly influence your own future ageing prospects by instituting such a regimen into your life, especially from fifty onwards.

Ageing, however, does not only involve physical and cognitive changes, it also can affect us emotionally or psychologically. Some of us rail against ageing, whilst others may learn to embrace it, despite the many challenges it presents. Still others may find themselves succumbing to the process of ageing and becoming overwhelmed by emotions of sadness and regret.

Most of our emotional difficulties with ageing relate to the world of loss and this will be a prime focus of our discussion, for ageing and loss, as Sheila will discover, are close friends, coming together like hand and glove. Let's explore some of the changes or losses that ageing introduces into our lives in greater details.

Physically, from as early as fifty onwards, men and women increasingly experience such changes. Both sexes are affected, albeit in different ways. Changes may be cosmetic due to alopecia or hair loss, hair thinning, loss of facial skin plasticity, reduced breast tissue and elasticity, loss of physical shape and weight gain in the wrong places due to hormonal changes, which are a normal part of ageing.

Physical changes can also impact on important bodily functions, from ED issues for men, lack of sexual drive in women, vaginal prolapse, reduction in bone density, reduced hearing and increasing use of glasses to assist with changes in the lens |of our eyes, to increasing forgetfulness due to our brains becoming easily distracted. The list goes on and on! It is unsurprising that ageing is sometimes described as not being for the faint-hearted.

All of these physical changes and losses come with an emotional price which varies from person to person. We will discuss these emotional responses later.

Then there are the multiple emotional losses that accompany increased ageing. For some of us, these can really mount up, with the loss of family members and close friends as time passes. It usually begins with the loss of parents, grandparents or siblings. On some occasions it may involve the loss of a child. Then, as the years pass, we increasingly lose close friends, siblings, spouses and long-term partners. Each death has an additive effect, building up a reservoir of grief.

There can also be other forms of loss. One of the most poignant is the arrival of dementia into a family or relationship. Since this condition is primarily an illness of ageing, encountering it can be a great challenge for those tasked with looking after anyone affected. For spouses or partners, often themselves senior citizens over seventy, this can be one of the saddest losses of all. For dementia gradually robs us of the person we have known and shared our lives with. This can be a devastating experience, as Sheila discovers.

Ageing can also highlight other losses. These may include those unfulfilled life dreams, broken relationships or separations, fractured relationships with adult children, the loss of independence created by the physical changes or illnesses associated with ageing, and finally the isolation and loneliness associated with the gradual loss of family and close friends to death.

The pragmatic approach to ageing involves firstly maintaining a sense of realism when dealing with the topic. There are no glib or easy solutions to many of the issues detailed above. Pragmatism would also point out that the experience of ageing can be incredibly different from one person to another, depending on a wide variety of factors. So, while some of us may have a really difficult time, others may find their journey less arduous. Pragmatism also teaches us that how we view and manage the trials of ageing will decide how emotionally distressed or not we will become when faced its challenge.

Pragmatism also teaches us to accept that whilst loss, grief, sadness and regret are a normal part of the ageing process, so, too, there will be times of great joy. These may include spending time with family, especially with grandchildren or close friends, engaging in activities you enjoy, taking pleasure in small everyday activities such as cooking or gardening, or becoming involved in social activities with others, etc.

Sheila's Story

Sheila is a retired journalist and the mother of two adult children, Trevor and Viv, and now a grandmother to two beautiful grandchildren. She has always hated the concept of ageing. Having reached the age of seventy, she finds that matters are not improving. Martin, her husband of forty-five years, who for three years has demonstrated signs of mild cognitive impairment, is eventually diagnosed with Alzheimer's disease, a common type of dementia. For Sheila, this is the final straw, the end of a long list of life losses, and she finds herself really struggling.

It begins in her late fifties, when she loses her older sister, Jenny, to a sudden brain haemorrhage. This is followed two years later by the loss of her mum, a chronic smoker, to lung cancer. She has always been able to pick up the phone and seek advice from her, and now this link is gone. Her dad died when she was in her teens, so her family is now reduced to a brother who lives in Spain and her sister Ruth, with whom she has always had a fractured relationship. She finds solace in her personal relationships with husband Martin, her two children, Trevor and Viv, and especially with close friends Kate and Amy.

Then, in her early sixties, her son Trevor, together with his wife and two grandchildren, move to New York, as he lands a job with a TV station. One of her main supports is gone. She particularly misses her two grandchildren. At the age of sixty-seven, one of her closest friends, Kate, develops breast cancer and following two years of extensive surgery, chemotherapy and radiotherapy finally succumbs to the illness. Sheila is with her, every step of this journey, and is grief-stricken following her death as they have been lifelong friends. She is overcome with sadness, emotional pain, regret and anger towards life, with her whole world shrinking by the second.

Ageing has affected Sheila in other ways, apart from the above. The menopause wasn't kind to her, and ever since she has struggled with her weight. She abhors the cosmetic issues (highlighted earlier) which accompany ageing. Her eyesight is a major annoyance, as she constantly both uses and loses her short- and long-distance glasses, leading to intense frustration. Her great fear is that this could deteriorate further, as reading is one of her main pastimes. She is also struggling with osteoarthritis of the right knee, which is interfering greatly with her mobility. Even her hearing, on the left side, is deteriorating. As she often joked with Kate before her death, she feels like an ageing car which is slowly packing in.

Between these physical changes, the loss of both her mum and best friend Kate, combined with the knowledge that her lifelong partner Martin is facing a slow descent into the abyss of dementia, Sheila becomes increasingly emotionally distressed. Normally she would turn to Martin for support and advice. Now she has to cope with the reality of ageing on her own. Sometimes the accumulated losses of the previous twenty years engulf her in a tsunami of negative emotions. She also refuses to engage the services of the system when coping with Martin, as she believes that this means she is letting him down. She prefers to go it alone.

Her daughter Viv assists her in any way she can, both emotionally and practically. She lives several hours away, however, so is of limited assistance to her. Sheila finds herself increasingly isolated, constantly crying and increasingly drawing on the support of her other close friend, Amy, whom she has also known for decades. Amy mentions that Sheila is struggling to cope emotionally and suggests that she might consider talking to a therapist friend before matters get any worse.

This proves to be an important step in Sheila's battle to come to terms with these multiple changes and losses, now threatening to overwhelm her. After a long discussion on the importance of grief and loss in relation to ageing, the therapist suggests some strategies, including our pragmatic blueprint, to assist her with her current difficulties. She finds this process extremely helpful.

These are Sheila's answers:

1. **How is this situation making me feel?**
    'My primary emotional responses to the changes and losses associated with ageing are sadness and regret.'

2. **What is it about this situation that is causing me to feel this way?**
    'I feel sadness because I have lost my mum, sister Jenny and closest friend Kate, all of them irreplaceable, and I am bereft without them.

    'I have also lost my son Trevor and grandchildren to emigration. Most of all it is the loss of my relationship with Martin, my bedrock, which is causing me the greatest sadness. It is so distressing to observe him gradually losing contact with everything around him. He is very frightened by this, and there is so little I can do to assist him.

'I know it is vanity but I am also sad at the loss of my looks, vigour, body shape, eyesight, even hearing over the past two decades.

'I also regret that Martin and I didn't do more together when he was well, and that I didn't do more to keep myself physically in better shape. There is also a longstanding sadness and regret that my sister Ruth and I have never been able to make up. So many years wasted.'

3. **What in my thinking is preventing me from dealing with this situation?**

'The main block to dealing with my sadness is my inability to come to terms with the loss of so many wonderful people from my life, together with my refusal to deal with the multiple physical and other changes associated with ageing.

'The main block to managing my regret is my refusal to accept that none of us can see into the future or predict what will happen and make decisions based on such predictions.'

4. **What in my behaviour is preventing me from dealing with this situation?**

'I know that I am not dealing with my emotions or the situation at the moment. In relation to Martin, I am not seeking assistance from others, especially the available services. I am making no effort in relation to my physical appearance or lifestyle and I am retreating into my shell and not engaging more with the community.'

5. **How can I short-circuit my thinking and behavioural blocks to deal more effectively with this situation?**

'I have to accept, following a chat with my therapist, that I am going through a natural grief process as a consequence of repeated losses of every type. I now understand that it is normal and healthy to feel extreme sadness, often coming in waves, and to cry on occasion if such feelings threaten to overwhelm me, as they often do. I have lost my sister, my mum and my friend Kate, together with the loss of my deep personal relationship with Martin, whom I love to bits. Being unable to share with him and seek out his advice is breaking my heart. I have also lost those wonderful years we could have had together.

'Ageing itself, I now realize, is characterized by a series of losses for each one of us and I am no different from anyone else. Realistically, there is no time frame to get over such losses, some of them excruciatingly painful. Grief is a process which may continue on for long periods, perhaps for life, but one that I will become better at managing and handling.

'In relation to my behaviour, there is much work to be done. I need to take matters in hand and work with a fitness coach to lose weight and become fitter. It's time to explore the idea of bifocals and a possible hearing aid. I need to return to caring for myself as well as everyone else. I must also investigate any community or other supports to draw upon for Martin, as his situation will gradually deteriorate over time. With Viv and Amy's assistance, it's time to engage more, socially, with the local community.'

Sheila then decides, together with her therapist, Amy and the support of her daughter, to put the above blueprint into action. Amy and Viv contact a fitness trainer to help her. With his assistance Sheila tackles her lifestyle, introducing some serious dietary and fitness regimens. Over a period of six months she becomes leaner and fitter, developing increased energy and zest for life. She moves to using varifocals and has a tiny hearing aid fitted into her glasses. These aids transform her life, and she notices herself becoming cognitively more alert.

She also contacts community services to assist with Martin. He begins to attend an Alzheimer's day care centre, three days a week. She makes new friends with many of the spouses who are also caring for loved ones with dementia and finds them to be a great support system. The years to come are not going to be easy, but she is slowly coming to terms with Martin's increasing loss of memory and cognitive function, together with the resultant loss of their special relationship. She cries regularly about this and for the loss of those who have passed on. She now accepts that this is normal and healthy, so she no longer tries to block it happening. She has developed other coping mechanisms, which include joining a book club, playing cards in the house with Amy and other friends, doing an online language course and taking up the guitar.

Sheila now accepts that ageing is inevitably associated with loss, that loss in turn is associated with natural emotions of sadness and regret, and that this is both normal and healthy. She has, however, learned how to adapt to the new situation in which she finds herself. It doesn't stop her admitting to Amy on a regular basis that ageing still sucks!

Death and Dying

It is fitting to end our journey by exploring the world of death and dying, something each one of us will encounter at some stage during our lives. Losing someone we love to death, or encountering a terminal illness in ourselves or someone close to us, are associated with profound periods of transitional change. Death can set loose a maelstrom of distressing emotions, especially sadness and regret.

The above situations lead us naturally into the world of grief, something I dealt with in my last book. Grief is a condition where we experience intense sorrow, sadness, emotional pain and heartache arising from the death of a loved one. It can also be triggered in advance when someone close to us is diagnosed with a terminal illness such as cancer or motor neurone disease. Both situations highlighted above are triggered by the loss of that precious person from our lives, for ever, and what might have been in the months and years that would have followed. There are also our natural emotional reactions to the profound changes that such a loss brings into our lives.

Another group who may experience the emotions associated with grief are those diagnosed with a terminal illness. They are now increasingly aware how their time with us is fast coming to an end. For many of those who experience this reality, loss in the form of a potential future can also lead to powerful emotions of sadness and regret. Such losses may include spending precious time with spouses, children, grandchildren or close friends in particular.

At the heart of the grief response in all three groups are the emotional reactions of sadness, regret and emotional pain, together with the challenges of responding to the enormous changes that death introduces into all of our lives.

In the case of losing a loved one, such as a spouse, parent or child, this change will involve learning how to manage changes in domestic and social circumstances, handling the silence created by their going and dealing with the loneliness which follows. All of this change is inevitably wrapped up in a cloak of sadness and pain.

If coming to terms with a terminal illness in someone we love, there are similar changes to be faced. The reality of their upcoming death. The enormous hole in our lives which their passing is going to create. In the short term there are a raft of immediate changes to be made in terms of palliative care and ensuring that loved ones are as comfortable as possible in their current surroundings. This may require significant interactions with palliative-care services and also the temporary suspension of your life as you know it, until the person you love has died. It can be a significant challenge to embrace such changes whilst carrying with you intense sadness and pain.

If you yourself have been diagnosed with a terminal illness, then life is now presenting you with the ultimate challenge and one that faces us all, namely the end of your life. In the Western world we are reluctant to contemplate the reality of our death. When and how will it happen? How well prepared am I? Where am I going to? What was my life really all about? What about those left behind? These are the kinds of questions which you are now faced with and also most likely struggling with.

There is probably a mixture of profound sadness and regret as you try to come to terms with the knowledge that your future in this world is slowly coming to an end. Some of you may have a strong spiritual base and be finding that your belief system is assisting you greatly in coming to terms with your situation. Or you may be agnostic, or have a humanistic base, and possibly in some cases finding the spectre of death more challenging.

This section is not going to offer you some unrealistic expectations that coming through such periods of change is going to be easy, or that there is a quick fix to dealing with either grief or a terminal illness and the emotional tsunami that both bring in their wake. The best you can do during such periods is to try to survive as best you can, and deal with the situation you find yourself in, in the most pragmatic manner possible. This will involve an acceptance that your life is never going to be the same, following any encounter with death or dying.

The pragmatic approach to death is that it is a reality for all of us, that it is inevitable and that coming to terms with our own mortality is perhaps one of the most important tasks each one of us must face. The death of a loved one, whether expected or, as is often the case, unexpected, is one of the greatest losses any of us will ever experience. Such a loss will be accompanied by long periods of profound sadness, emotional pain and regret. There is no time frame set in stone for such a period to end. Their death is going to punch a major hole in our lives and that hole will never be filled. We are going to experience significant changes in our personal, social and domestic worlds, to which we will have to gradually adapt.

How can you adapt a pragmatic approach to your own death, if you are diagnosed with a terminal illness? This seems to be a daunting task. I have walked this road with many wonderful people throughout my career and they have shown me that it is indeed possible. This often involves an acceptance of the reality of your upcoming death and a decision to make the best of each day left to you. Most of all, deciding that you will focus on making sure that you assist those who will be left behind, as much as humanly possible, to deal with your upcoming departure from this life.

In all of the above distressing situations, a pragmatic approach can assist you to recognize that while there is little you can do to change the reality of the death, or upcoming death, of a loved one, or of your own impending death, you can do much to change how you view such situations and hopefully somehow reduce the emotional distress which usually follows in their wake.

Now let's meet Damien, whose story will reverberate in the hearts of many readers. His life irrevocably changes when death, in the form of his mum succumbing to Covid-19, enters his life. Then, just as he is struggling with the mountain of grief due to her passing, his brother is diagnosed with terminal cancer.

Damien's Story

Damien is a forty-four-year-old engineer who has so far remained relatively unscathed by the winds and storms of life. He is married to Megan, who works as a pharmacist, and they have two small children. His life, as one would expect from an engineer, is completely structured, organized and routine. He is a man who doesn't do emotions well. In this he takes after his father, who had been a remote figure in his childhood.

Then life comes roaring in. Covid-19 begins to wreck his normal daily routines, with Megan and himself both struggling to adapt to all of the changes the virus introduces into their lives. Working from home combined with home schooling taxes them both to the hilt. But worse is to come, a lot worse!

Damien's mother Irene, in her early sixties, a fit and healthy woman, begins to show symptoms of Covid-19. Initially she seems to be managing, but then five days later her condition suddenly deteriorates. She is rushed into hospital and within hours is on a ventilator. Damien, who has always been especially close to his mother, now faces the reality that he cannot go in to see her or hold her hand or be with her. Due to public-health constraints he had forgone the chance to visit her in the early stages of her illness and is now filled with regret about this. It all happened so quickly. His dad is now left cocooning at home as a result of his wife's diagnosis. Damien has two younger brothers, Mike who lives abroad and Andy who lives close by.

His mum, whom he loves to bits, is now alone, in the ICU, on a ventilator, surrounded by nurses and doctors, all encased in PPE. Damien, who rarely shows any emotion, breaks down in front of Megan when the hospital gently informs him that his mum is seriously ill and unlikely to make it.

Finally, he receives the phone call that all families dread, where the ICU nurses advise the family that if Andy or himself wishes to say goodbye to Irene they will allow one or the other a final opportunity to do so. As the eldest, Damien is the one chosen. He dons protective gear and visits his mum for the last time. His heart is breaking that he cannot hold or embrace her. It is one of the most devastating experiences of his previously sheltered life.

Within hours of this visit, his mum dies and another nightmare begins. He is informed by the funeral director that his mum cannot be waked in the traditional sense, where her body would be laid out embalmed in an open coffin at home, for twenty-four hours or so, for family, loved ones and close friends to pay their respects. Nor can there be a normal church service or burial as only ten people in total, including the celebrant, will be allowed to attend both. Damien and Andy are totally devastated, as is his dad, who is almost beside himself with grief. His dad is especially distressed at not being able to accompany Irene, his wife and lifelong partner, on her final journey. His brother Mike is also distressed as he is unable to travel due to Covid-19 restrictions. How will any of them ever come to terms with such a loss and in such circumstances?

The funeral and burial that follow are one of the most surreal experiences of Damien's life. There are no embraces or handshakes, no rejoicing about the life of a woman who had given everything to her family and society, no proper church service for a committed believer, which she had been, no live music, no procession of family, friends and colleagues to the cemetery and finally only a short service at the grave. Then their mum is gone from them for ever. All that they are left with are memories.

For Damien, the months which follow are horrendous. He tries desperately to block out the waves of sadness, emotional pain and regret. Despite his best efforts, he constantly breaks down into tears, often at the most inappropriate times. He tries to focus solely on staying busy, and thankfully his job allows him to continue doing so. But the memories of what happened keep recurring and with them floods of tears. He visits the grave regularly, finding some solace there. He attempts to focus on looking after his dad, struggling to cope with his grief on top of his own, and finds himself increasingly emotionally overwhelmed. Although close to his brothers, especially Andy, he still struggles to share his emotional difficulties with either of them.

Six months later, he is slowly beginning to come to terms with the reality that his mum is truly gone. That he will never see her again in this life. Then the next bombshell arrives. His youngest brother Andy rings him with the news that he has been diagnosed with advanced pancreatic cancer and given a short period to live, probably in the region of eight to ten weeks. He had presented to his family doctor with jaundice. Following scans and other tests, his condition is diagnosed as terminal. Andy is more upset that he is leaving behind a partner and two small children than about his own upcoming demise.

Damien now finds himself on a different journey with Andy, whose care is shared with the local palliative-care team. There is little to be done surgically and he has chosen to forsake palliative chemotherapy as he believes that it will just make him feel miserable for his few remaining weeks or months. Andy, after some initial emotions of anger and depression, is now acceptant of his diagnosis, spending most of his time trying to ensure that his wife and children are emotionally coping and financially secure, and so he keeps up a brave face for them.

He does not have his mum's strong faith but is quite pragmatic about his upcoming death. As he good-humouredly reveals to Damien, he is unsure what lies beyond the grave and has always been agnostic about religion. But when he leaves this world, he is happy that he has lived a good life and always tried to help others, so if God does exist, he would be happy to meet him. If on the other hand there is nothing after death, then he would no longer be around to worry about it.

Meanwhile Damien simply cannot accept that he is going to lose a second person whom he loves dearly, in such a short period of time. His emotions are all over the place, as he is already grieving for his mum and now beginning to grieve for Andy. His emotions range from sadness at the thought of his brother's death, to regret that he has not spent more time with him, to anger at life, to depression, as he somehow feels that he has let Andy down. He is also increasingly anxious about having to go through the same funeral regimen as with Irene. He is also concerned that Andy might suffer, the closer he approaches his time. He is struggling to see any future without Andy and his mum. How will he be able to continue on? How will he survive such a period of change? How will his dad survive this awful time? Will his dad be next?

The only thing keeping him going is the importance of keeping up a brave face for Andy and his family, and also the love of his wife Megan. Fleeting thoughts of joining his mum, when Andy is gone, keep intruding into his mind, but he knows that would only destroy the lives of those he loves, so he dismisses them.

Megan becomes increasingly concerned at his emotional state, recognizing that he is still grieving for his mum while trying to be there for Andy. She notices how he is withdrawing more and refusing to discuss either situation with her. While aware that much of what he is feeling is to be expected, Megan still dreads what will happen when Andy dies. She persuades Damien to visit a therapist to assist him with the grief process. This turns out to be a wise decision as he finds the therapist empathetic and easy to talk to.

His therapist explains the grief process to him. How overwhelming the emotions of sadness, regret, anxiety, depression and anger can be. How there is no time limit on these emotions. How changed his life is going to be as a result of his mum's passing and Andy's upcoming death. She also warns how, when presented with a loved one's terminal diagnosis, as in the case of Andy, our emotional mind can block us from dealing with the emotions of sadness, emotional pain and regret, which the death of his mum has already begun to trigger. She suggests using our pragmatic blueprint as a tool to explore his current situation further and Damien finds this process really helpful.

These are Damien's answers:

1. **How is this situation making me feel?**
    'Losing mum to Covid-19 combined with the approaching death of Andy has triggered emotions of sadness, emotional pain and regret.'

2. **What is it about this situation that is causing me to feel this way?**
    'I feel sadness because my mum is gone and I feel intensely the loss of her warmth, kindness and total love for us all. I have also lost all those years to come, where she could have shared the lives of her grandchildren, watching them grow up into young adults. I am also gutted for my dad, who will struggle to keep going without her. The thought that I will never again see her smile, embrace her, or share my ups and downs with her leaves me feeling lonely and intensely sad.

    'I also feel sad that I am now going to lose Andy. I am gutted for his wife and children, who are going to miss him so much. He is not only my brother, but also my best friend, someone I could always discuss things with. Now that, too, will be gone.

'I feel regret because of the manner in which my mum died. That she had to die alone, and go through the awfulness of being buried in the manner in which she was, without her family, friends and community accompanying her on her last journey.

'I also feel sadness and regret that Andy will have to go through the same process, made even more complex as he has expressed a wish to be cremated. There is also some regret that I did not spend more time with him. If only I had known that he was going to leave us so soon.'

3. **What in my thinking is preventing me from dealing with this situation?**

    'The main block to dealing with my sadness is my inability to come to terms with the loss of my mum and accept that she is truly gone and will not be coming back in this life. I am also not accepting that it is normal to feel such emotions, and that they may continue for a longer period than I assumed. So too with Andy. I am struggling to come to terms with the reality that he, too, will soon be gone from us, in a similar manner to that of my mum.

    'In relation to my regret, the main block is my struggle to forgive myself for not anticipating that either my mum or Andy were going to die and that I would have preferred to have spent more time with them. I am also struggling to forgive myself for the manner in which we had to bury my mum.'

4. **What in my behaviour is preventing me from dealing with this situation?**

    'I am withdrawing from everyone, especially Megan, and refusing to discuss how I feel with her, or with Mike or other good friends. I am drinking more on my own, which is not healthy. It cannot be healthy either to suppress tears when they suddenly come bubbling up.'

5. **How can I short-circuit my thinking and behavioural blocks to deal more effectively with this situation?**

    'I have to accept, following my chat with my therapist, that what I am going through is a natural grief process. It is normal and healthy to feel sadness, often coming in waves, and to cry on occasion if such feelings become overwhelming, as they frequently do. The reason for my sadness is obvious, the permanent loss of my mum, whom I loved so dearly and who was the centre of my life for so long. I have to accept that this grief process is going to be there for the long haul, perhaps years, and that these waves of sadness and other emotions will be constant companions. I have to adjust to the changes which Mum's death have also introduced into my life. The silence, not being able to see or hear her, having to take care of Dad on my own, the disappearance of those wonderful family occasions of which she was the conductor and those multiple everyday cameos to do with her being present.

    'I am also already starting to grieve for Andy and his approaching death. I am grieving for the loss of his future, too, which his family and I are going to miss out on. This is going to take a long time to get over, if ever.

'It is natural to have some regrets about the manner in which my mum both died and was laid to rest, as will be the case with Andy, but there is little that I can do to change the situation. It is the situation which is abnormal, not me, so I must learn to let this go.

'Finally, I need to make some changes in my behaviours, stop drinking and comfort eating, share more with Megan, my therapist and others, stop withdrawing from everyone and accept that this is going to be a tough period for us all. It is going to be hard but we will survive and come out the other side.'

Let's now discover what happens when Damien decides, following this pragmatic analysis and with his therapist's and Megan's assistance, to put the above blueprint into action.

He begins with his behaviour, cutting out the alcohol and food binges, talking and sharing more with Megan and his therapist and allowing himself to cry in a normal way when grief overwhelms him. He also begins to plan with Andy's wife how best to celebrate his life, in both the time remaining and for the services afterwards. After some online discussions with neighbours, for example, it is decided that when Andy dies, everyone will silently line the street, in a socially distanced manner, in a powerful show of affection and respect for both him and his family and sharing with them in their grief. This is what happens when Andy dies six weeks later.

Damien now accepts that the sadness will be with him long-term and that he has to go wherever his grief journey takes him in relation to both his mum and Andy. He also recognizes that his life will never be the same again with their loss. It will be different and he will have to discover a new path. But as he discusses with his therapist, this is the reality of life. There will always be periods of change like this, some of which are distressing beyond belief. Alongside countless others in his position, he will have to learn new ways of adapting and moving on with his life. New ways to heal.

CONCLUSION

One of the great privileges accorded to family doctors such as myself, especially those who have cared from birth to death for multiple generations, is that of walking the walk with so many special, wonderful people as we struggle to come to terms with the challenges and vicissitudes of life. The plethora of periods of transitional change presented in this book are but a microcosm of such challenges.

It is extremely likely that you have recognized yourself in many of the stories and life situations discussed. If not, then it is only a question to time before one of them arrives into your life. We cannot escape from the harsh realities of life or from the challenges which such periods of change will present to us as individual human beings.

Rather than railing against such times, it is healthier to find another way of managing them. I hope that the pragmatic blueprint presented in this book will have given you a road map to chart your way safely through them.

Change can seriously challenge your emotional resilience, your capacity to cope with the slings and arrows of life. You have two choices when problematic situations arise: find yourself engulfed by negative emotions and behaviours, or try instead to pragmatically problem-solve them. One road leads to emotional distress, the other to a healthier philosophical understanding that life is not going to adapt to suit you, so you have to adapt to it. This second road leads to inner peace.

It is key, when applying our pragmatic blueprint to your life, that you are kind to yourself. Accept that you will regularly get it wrong, mess up, fail, but you will get up and keep going, and that you, like me, are not perfect and never will be. You will often find yourself stumbling along a road full of potholes, sometimes in the dark, unsure where life is leading you. For uncertainty is the cornerstone of change. Pragmatism will save you at such times. If you are also more self-acceptant of yourself for the beautiful, unique, human person that you are, but learn to take active responsibility for your actions, then it becomes much easier to be pragmatic when a period of distressing change arrives.

If you can learn to adapt and embrace change and allow it to deepen both your understanding of yourself and of life, then you will become truly resilient. This is my wish for each of you.

BIBLIOGRAPHY

Introduction

Barry, H.P. (2017). *Emotional Resilience: How to Safeguard your Mental Health.* Orion Spring. London.

1. The Many Faces of Change

Barry, H.P. (2009). *Flagging the Therapy: Pathways out of Depression and Anxiety.* Liberties Press. Dublin.

Barry, H.P. (2017). *Emotional Resilience: How to Safeguard your Mental Health.* Orion Spring. London.

Barry, H.P. (2018). *Self-Acceptance: How to Banish the Self-Esteem Myth, Accept Yourself Unconditionally and Revolutionize your Mental Health.* Orion Spring. London.

Barry, H.P. (2020). *Emotional Healing: How to Put Yourself Back Together Again.* Orion Spring. London.

Darwin, C. (1859). *On the Origin of Species by Means of Natural Selection, or the Preservation of Favoured Races in the Struggle for Life.* John Murray. London.

Davidson, R.J. & Begley, S. (2013). *The Emotional Life of your Brain – How to Change the Way you Think, Feel and Live.* Hodder and Stoughton. London.

2. Embracing Change

Barry, H.P. (2009). *Flagging the Therapy: Pathways out of Depression and Anxiety.* Liberties Press. Dublin.

Barry, H.P. (2017). *Emotional Resilience: How to Safeguard your Mental Health.* Orion Spring. London.

Ellis, A. (1962). *Reason and Emotion in Psychotherapy.* Lyle Stuart. New York.

Ellis, A. (1996). *Better, Deeper and More Enduring Brief Therapy. The Rational Emotive Behavior Therapy Approach.* Brunner/ Mazel, Inc. New York.

3. Why Change Can Make You Anxious

Barry, H.P. (2009). *Flagging the Therapy: Pathways out of Depression and Anxiety.* Liberties Press. Dublin.

Barry, H.P. (2016). *Anxiety and Panic: How to Reshape your Anxious Mind and Brain.* Liberties Press. Dublin.

Barry, H.P. (2017). *Emotional Resilience: How to Safeguard your Mental Health.* Orion Spring. London.

Barry, H.P. (2018). *Self-Acceptance: How to Banish the Self-Esteem Myth, Accept Yourself Unconditionally and Revolutionize your Mental Health.* Orion Spring. London.

Murphy, E. (2013). *Five Steps to Happiness.* Liberties Press. Dublin.

4. How to Manage Your 'Change' Anxiety

Barry, H.P. (2016). *Anxiety and Panic: How to Reshape your Anxious Mind and Brain.* Liberties Press. Dublin.

Barry, H.P. (2017). *Emotional Resilience: How to Safeguard your Mental Health.* Orion Spring. London.

Barry, H.P. (2018). *Self-Acceptance: How to Banish the Self-Esteem Myth, Accept Yourself Unconditionally and Revolutionize your Mental Health.* Orion Spring. London.

Barry, H.P. (2020*). Emotional Healing: How to Put Yourself Back Together Again.* Orion Spring. London.

Santoro, N., Epperson, C.N. & Mathews, S.B. (2015). 'Menopausal Symptoms and Their Management'. *Endocrinol Metab Clin North Am.* 44(3):497–515.

5. Why Change Can Make You Frustrated

Abbasi, I.S. & Alghamdi, N.G. (2015). 'The Prevalence, Predictors, Causes, Treatments, and Implications of Procrastination Behaviors in General, Academic, and Work Setting'. *International Journal of Psychological Studies.* 7(1).

Barry, H.P. (2017). *Emotional Resilience: How to Safeguard your Mental Health.* Orion Spring. London.

Wilde, J. (2012). 'The Relationship between Frustration Intolerance and Academic Achievement in College'. *International Journal of Higher Education.* 1(2).

6. How to Manage Your 'Change' Frustration

Barry, H.P. (2017). *Emotional Resilience: How to Safeguard your Mental Health.* Orion Spring. London.

Fingerman, K.L. (2017). 'Millennials and Their Parents: Implications of the New Young Adulthood for Midlife Adults'. *Innov Aging*. 1(3).

Jung, J.I., Son, J.S., Kim, Y.O., et al (2018). 'Changes of depression and job stress in workers after merger without downsizing'. *Ann of Occup and Environ Med*. 30: 54.

7. Why Change Can Make You Depressed

Barry, H.P. (2009). *Flagging the Therapy: Pathways out of Depression and Anxiety*. Liberties Press. Dublin.

Barry, H.P. (2012). *Depression: A Practical Guide*. Liberties Press. Dublin.

Barry, H.P. (2017). *Emotional Resilience: How to Safeguard your Mental Health*. Orion Spring. London.

Barry, H.P. (2018). *Self-Acceptance: How to Banish the Self-Esteem Myth, Accept Yourself Unconditionally and Revolutionize your Mental Health*. Orion Spring. London.

Barry, H.P. (2020). *Emotional Healing: How to Put Yourself Back Together Again*. Orion Spring. London.

8. How to Manage Your 'Change' Depression

Barry, H.P. (2009). *Flagging the Therapy: Pathways out of Depression and Anxiety*. Liberties Press. Dublin.

Barry, H.P. (2012). *Depression: A Practical Guide*. Liberties Press. Dublin.

Barry, H.P. (2017). *Emotional Resilience: How to Safeguard your Mental Health*. Orion Spring. London.

Barry, H.P. (2018). *Self-Acceptance: How to Banish the Self-Esteem Myth, Accept Yourself Unconditionally and Revolutionize your Mental Health.* Orion Spring. London.

Barry, H.P. (2020). *Emotional Healing: How to Put Yourself Back Together Again.* Orion Spring.

Javadifar, N., Majlesi, F., Nikbakht, A., Nedjat, S. & Montazeri, A. (2016). 'Journey to Motherhood in the First Year After Child Birth'. *Journal of family & reproductive health.* 10(3), 146–153.

Kaltenboeck, A. & Harmer, C. (2018). 'The neuroscience of depressive disorders: A brief review of the past and some considerations about the future.' *Brain and Neuroscience Advances.* 2: 1–6.

Kubicek, B., Korunka, C., Raymo, J. M. & Hoonakker, P. (2011). Psychological well-being in retirement: the effects of personal and gendered contextual resources. *Journal of occupational health psychology.* 16(2), 230–246.

Lau, K.K.H., et al. (2019). 'Examining the Effects of Couples' Real-Time Stress and Coping Processes on Interaction Quality: Language Use as a Mediator'. *Frontiers in Psychology.* 9: 2598.

9. Why Change Can Make You Feel Hurt

Barry, H.P. (2009). *Flagging the Therapy: Pathways out of Depression and Anxiety.* Liberties Press. Dublin.

Barry, H.P. (2017). *Emotional Resilience: How to Safeguard your Mental Health.* Orion Spring. London.

Barry, H.P. (2020). *Emotional Healing: How to Put Yourself Back Together Again.* Orion Spring. London.

Tchalova, K. & Eisenberger, N.I. (2015). 'How the Brain Feels the Hurt of Heartbreak: Examining the Neurobiological Overlap Between Social and Physical Pain'. In: Arthur W. Toga, editor. *Brain Mapping: An Encyclopaedic Reference.* 3: 15–20. Academic Press: Elsevier.

Leary, M.R. (2015). Emotional responses to interpersonal rejection. *Dialogues in clinical neuroscience.* 17(4): 435–441.

10. How to Manage Your 'Change' Hurt

Barry, H.P. (2009). *Flagging the Therapy: Pathways out of Depression and Anxiety.* Liberties Press. Dublin.

Barry, H.P. (2017). *Emotional Resilience: How to Safeguard your Mental Health.* Orion Spring. London.

Barry, H.P. (2020). *Emotional Healing: How to Put Yourself Back Together Again.* Orion Spring. London.

Moles, R.L. & Leventhal J.M. (2014). 'Sexual Abuse and Assault in Children and Teens: Time to Prioritize Prevention'. *Journal of Adolescent Health.* 55(3): 312–313.

Pheko, M.M., Monteiro, M. & Segopolo, M.T. (2017). 'When work hurts: A conceptual framework explaining how organizational culture may perpetuate workplace bullying'. *Journal of Human Behaviour in the Social Environment.* 27(6): 571–588.

11. Why Change Can Make You Ashamed

Barry, H.P. (2018). *Self-Acceptance: How to Banish the Self-Esteem Myth, Accept Yourself Unconditionally and Revolutionize your Mental Health.* Orion Spring. London.

Barry, H.P. (2020). *Emotional Healing: How to Put Yourself Back Together Again.* Orion Spring. London.

12. How to Manage Your 'Change' Shame

American Cancer Society (2019). Breast Cancer Facts & Figures 2019–2020. *Atlanta: American Cancer Society, Inc.*

Barry, H.P. (2018). *Self-Acceptance: How to Banish the Self-Esteem Myth, Accept Yourself Unconditionally and Revolutionize your Mental Health.* Orion Spring. London.

Barry, H.P. (2020). *Emotional Healing: How to Put Yourself Back Together Again.* Orion Spring. London.

Candea, D-M. & Szentagotai, A. (2013). 'Shame and psychopathology: from research to clinical practice'. *Journal of Cognitive and Behavioural Psychotherapies.* 13(1): 97–109.

Cunningham, K.C., LoSavio, S.T., Dennis P.A., et al. (2019). 'Shame as a mediator between posttraumatic stress disorder symptoms and suicidal ideation among veterans.' *J Affect Disorder.* 243: 216–219.

Hack, J. & Martin, J. (2018). 'Expressed Emotion, Shame, and Non-Suicidal Self-Injury.' *Int. J. Environ. Res. Public Health.* 15(5): 890.

Klik, K.A., Williams, S.L. & Reynolds, K.J. (2019). 'Toward understanding mental illness stigma and help-seeking: A social identity perspective.' *Soc Sci Med.* 222: 35–43.

Leary, M.R. (2015). Emotional responses to interpersonal rejection. *Dialogues in clinical neuroscience.* 17(4): 435–441.

Velotti, P., Garofalo, C., Bottazzi, F. & Caretti V. (2017). 'Faces of Shame: Implications for Self-Esteem, Emotion

Regulation, Aggression, and Well-Being'. *The Journal of Psychology*. 151(2): 171–184.

13. Why Change Can Trigger Sadness and Regret

Barry, H.P. (2020). *Emotional Healing: How to Put Yourself Back Together Again*. Orion Spring. London.

Bonanno, G.A. (2009). *The other side of sadness: What the new science of bereavement tells us about life after loss*. Basic Books. New York.

14. How to Manage Your 'Change' Sadness and Regret

Al Ubaidi, B.A. (2017). 'Empty nest syndrome: pathway to 'destruction or construction'. *J Fam Med Dis Prev*. 3: 064.

Barry, H.P. (2020). *Emotional Healing: How to Put Yourself Back Together Again*. Orion Spring. London.

Hamczyk, M.R., Nevado, R.M., Baretinno, A., Fuster, V. & Andres, V. (2020). 'Biological Versus Chronological Vascular Aging'. *JACC*. 75(8).

Kübler-Ross, E. (1969). *On Death and Dying*. Macmillan. New York.

Kübler-Ross, E. & Kessler, D. (2005). *On Grief and Grieving: Finding the Meaning of Grief Through the Five Stages of Loss*. Scribner. New York.

Kyota, A. & Kanda, K. (2019). 'How to come to terms with facing death: a qualitative study examining the experiences of patients with terminal cancer'. *BMC Palliat Care*. 18(1): 33.

Mount, S.D. & Moas, S. (2015). 'Re-purposing the "empty nest".' *Journal of Family Psychotherapy*. 26(3): 247–252.

Razai, M.S. (2018). 'Patient Experiences of Terminal Illness Toward the End of Life: A Reflective Narrative Report'. *J Patient Exp*. 5(4): 279–281.

INDEX

Index

belief systems 27–9, 43, 48, 73,
    125–6
biological age v. chronological age
    250–2
bipolar disorder 223
bitterness 81, 104, 175, 178–9,
    186, 199
blogging 233
blues, having the 125
brain
    developing 193
    and emotions 18–21, 32
'brain-dead' 144, 148
'brain fog' 12
break-ups, relationship 79–80,
    153–61, 184–5, 238
breast cancer 224–34, 253

cancer 224–34
    positive thinking and 29
    stigma and 225, 229
    terminal 253, 262, 265–7
care, long-term nursing 171–5
careers, turning pastimes into
    14–15
cascading 51
catastrophizing 50–1, 52, 63, 74,
    82
CBT (Cognitive Behaviour
    Therapy) 27, 29, 218
challenge, of change 15–17
chemotherapy 226, 228
children

abused 192
acute illness and 16
adult 102–8
the baby question 79, 114–21,
    153
becoming a parent 142–53
break-ups and 153–5, 157
moving away 244–9
rating your 130
siblings 170–83, 197–8, 253
chocolate 92
chronological age v. biological age
    250–2
climate change 13
Cognitive Behaviour Therapy
    (CBT) 27, 29, 218
'Coin Exercise' (*Emotional
    Resilience*) 50
consequence, behavioural 25–6
control, being in 49–50
Covid-19 pandemic 69–72, 72–7,
    262–70
    ageing and 249
    frustration 90–1
    panic-buying 25
    speed of change 11, 13
creativity 14–15, 103

Damien's Story (death and dying)
    262–70
Darwin, Charles, *On the Origin of
    Species* 10
death

Index

Index

Index

ACKNOWLEDGEMENTS

I would like to start, as always, by thanking my editorial team at Orion UK for all their wonderful assistance in publishing this book. I want to especially thank my publishing editor, Pippa Wright, who has been so supportive in relation to this book. I am especially indebted to senior editor Ru Merritt for her invaluable support, assistance and advice – all of which greatly enhanced this manuscript. I would also like to thank Georgia Goodall for assisting me so ably in putting it all together. I am also indebted to publicist Francesca Pearce at Orion UK, and here in Ireland to publicity director Elaine Egan and Siobhan Tierney from Hachette Ireland for their assistance in the PR, sales and marketing areas during these difficult times. What a great team to have as an author!

I also owe a huge debt of gratitude to Vanessa Fox O'Loughlin, my agent, who made this whole project possible.

I would like to especially thank my dear friend and colleague Dr Muiris Houston of the *Irish Times* for taking the time to review the text, and for his friendship and support.

I send the warmest of thanks as always to my good friend Cathy Kelly (bestselling author and UNICEF ambassador) for her constant kindness and support throughout the years. I so value her encouragement and advice. I am also indebted to my dear friend and national treasure, Sr Stan, founder of Focus Ireland and The Sanctuary; she is a light in the darkness at times like this.

I am also deeply indebted to eminent Professor Ian Robertson, professor of psychology at Trinity College Dublin, and psychologist Fiona Doherty for taking the time to review the script and for their constant support and encouragement.

I would also like to warmly thank *Sunday Independent* columnist Stefanie Preissner for her support, and for taking the time to review *Embracing Change*. A special thanks to Dr Sabina Brennan, health psychologist, neuroscientist and author of *Beating Brain Fog*, and to Helen Downes, CEO of Shannon Chamber of Commerce, for taking time out of their busy schedules to review the book.

I am also so appreciative to my international colleagues Professor Ray Lam at University of British Columbia, Canada, and Professor Larry Culpepper at Boston University, USA – both of whom have been so supportive and took the time to review this book.

I would also like to thank the *Today With Clare Byrne* radio show, especially Clare herself (a real lady), together with her wonderful team – the excellent series producer Alistair O' Connell, producer Cora Ennis and so many others – for allowing my colleague Anne-Marie Creaven and I the opportunity to highlight key areas of mental health.

I say a special thanks to my sons Daniel and Joseph, Joseph's wife Sue and my beautiful granddaughter Saoirse, and to my daughter Lara, her husband Hans and my two much-loved grandsons Ciaran and Sean for all their love and support and for keeping me well grounded! We have had to truly embrace change during these difficult times, which have tested all of our resilience. Yet love, as always, has sustained us.

Acknowledgements

I reserve my biggest 'thank you' for my wife, Brenda, whose love, friendship, support, encouragement and particularly patience have made this book, and indeed the whole series, possible. You will always have my back as I have yours. You are my light in the darkness, and truly my soulmate. 'Mo ghra, mo chroi.' (My love, my heart).

ABOUT THE AUTHOR

Dr Harry Barry is a highly respected Irish author and medic, with over three decades of experience as a GP. With a keen interest in the area of mental health and suicide prevention, Dr Barry is the bestselling author of numerous books addressing various aspects of mental health, including anxiety, depression and toxic stress.

A practical guide to coping with trauma, loss and grief.

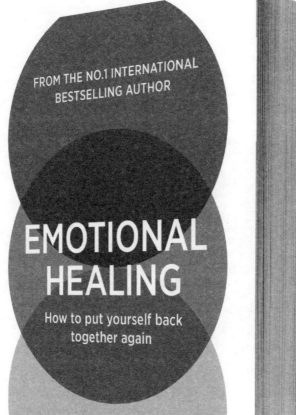

FROM THE NO.1 INTERNATIONAL
BESTSELLING AUTHOR

EMOTIONAL
HEALING

How to put yourself back
together again

DR HARRY BARRY

S

A practical guide to understanding and overcoming low self-esteem and self-doubt.

How to banish the self-esteem myth, accept yourself unconditionally and revolutionize your mental health.

SELF-ACCEPTANCE

DR HARRY BARRY

THE No.1 INTERNATIONAL BESTSELLING AUTHOR

S

A practical guide teaching you how
to best tackle life's challenges.

'Another masterpiece
from a cutting-edge expert'
Dr Muiris Houston,
The Irish Times

EMOTIONAL
RESILIENCE

How to safeguard your
mental health

THE BRAND NEW BOOK FROM
INTERNATIONAL BESTSELLING AUTHOR

DR HARRY BARRY

S

A practical guide to identifying and
managing stress.

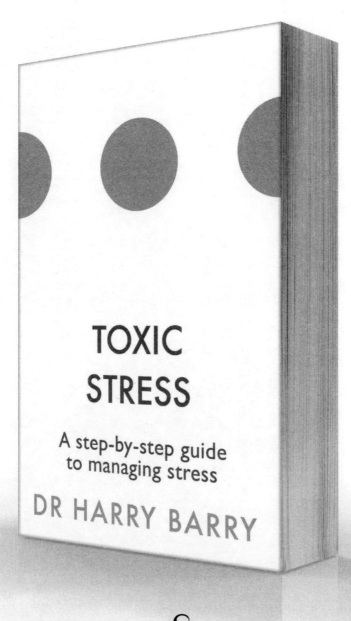

TOXIC
STRESS

A step-by-step guide
to managing stress

DR HARRY BARRY

S

A practical guide exploring the role of therapy in depression and anxiety.

FLAGGING THE THERAPY

Pathways out of depression and anxiety

DR HARRY BARRY

S

A practical guide to understanding and coping with anxiety, depression, addiction and suicide.

FLAGGING THE PROBLEM

A new approach to mental health

DR HARRY BARRY

S

A practical, four step programme to help you
understand and cope with depression.

DEPRESSION

A practical guide

DR HARRY BARRY

S

A practical guide to understanding, managing and overcoming anxiety and panic attacks.

ANXIETY AND PANIC

How to reshape your anxious mind and brain

DR HARRY BARRY

S